UNDERSTAND YOUR BACKACHE

A GUIDE TO
PREVENTION, TREATMENT, AND RELIEF

UNDERSTAND YOUR BACKACHE

A GUIDE TO
PREVENTION, TREATMENT, AND RELIEF

RENE CAILLIET, M.D.

Director of Rehabilitation Services
Santa Monica Hospital Medical Center
Santa Monica, California
and
Professor and Chairman (Retired)
Department of Rehabilitative Medicine
University of Southern California School of Medicine
Los Angeles, California

Illustrations by R. Cailliet, M.D.

F. A. DAVIS COMPANY Philadelphia

Also by Rene Cailliet:

FOOT AND ANKLE PAIN
HAND PAIN AND IMPAIRMENT
KNEE PAIN AND DISABILITY
LOW BACK PAIN SYNDROME
NECK AND ARM PAIN
SCOLIOSIS: DIAGNOSIS AND MANAGEMENT
THE SHOULDER IN HEMIPLEGIA
SHOULDER PAIN
SOFT TISSUE PAIN AND DISABILITY

Sixth printing 1992
Printed in the United States of America

Library of Congress Cataloging in Publication Data

Cailliet, Rene.
    Understand your backache.

    Includes index.
    1. Backache. I. Title.
RD768.C35 1984   617'.56   83-24071
ISBN 0-8036-1647-3

Preface

In this book, *Understand Your Backache*, I have attempted to explain *how* the lumbar spine functions, *where* in the tissues of the spine pain can result, and *how* improper movement or position of the spine can irritate these tissues and cause pain. Diagnosis based on appreciating *the* improper movement or position and understanding *the* specific tissue involved is discussed. Treatment of acute and recurrent low back pain and of chronic low back pain is discussed, with an explanation of *why* a particular treatment is helpful and what its purpose is.

Terms that are frequently used by physicians and therapists and even by daily publications are clarified and simplified so as to be clearly understood by the person who suffers from low back pain.

Two types of characters illustrate the text. The *workmen* are our friends and helpers and point out the normal tissues and functions. The *devil* points out the site of, cause of, and reason for pain. A picture tells more than the printed word. I hope that this presentation, fully supported by these drawings, helps the patient understand his or her low backache.

RENE CAILLIET, M.D.

Contents

*Denotes therapeutic exercise

Illustrations

xi

Introduction

Millions of patients have low back pain, and billions of dollars are spent treating low back pain. Numerous forms of tests are advocated to discover the cause of a particular low back pain. Many types of treatment, performed by many different types of physicians, therapists, or specialists, are claimed to be effective. Hundreds of terms bandied about by physicians and therapists are poorly understood, not understood at all, or thoroughly misunderstood.

Patients are labeled, branded, and classified, and they frequently become confused. Treatments are recommended but not explained. Other treatments are criticized. Symptoms are felt by patients and described to unhearing physicians. Doctors explain, but often in vague terms not clear to themselves and certainly less clear to the patients.

There must be an answer or answers. Certainly, there are numerous questions. Although much information regarding low back pain remains unknown, many aspects of low back pain are understood.

The person suffering from low back pain is entitled to know why he or she is suffering: where the pain originates, what causes it, and why a specific treatment is recommended for it.

Many books have been and will be written regarding low back pain. Most are biased by the physician's or therapist's training or personal experience and thus advocate *that* opinion and *that* approach. Surgeons are trained to operate and thus recommend surgery. Orthopedists claim that the back consists of bone and joints and therefore an orthopedic surgeon must operate. Neurosurgeons claim nerves are involved in the production of pain, so a neurosurgeon must diagnose and operate.

Tests are frequently the basis of diagnosis and treatment, but it must be remembered that *it is the patient who hurts* and must be treated, *not the test.*

Each test has its advocates who believe it to be "*the* most specific diagnostic test." Electromyographic experts extol the E.M.G., whereas radiol-

1

ogists acclaim diagnosis by x-rays. Orthopedists and neurosurgeons dispute these assertions and claim that it is within their expertise to interpret x-rays and CAT scans.

Physical therapists and exercise advocates expound on the value of exercise but disagree among themselves as to the concept and approach of a specific exercise. Whether the low back should be flexed (bent forward) or extended (arched) is the latest controversy. Both approaches may be right or wrong depending on the patient's specific problem, and while the argument rages, the patient is left in a quandary.

A treatment that is advocated must have an ultimate rationale, a reason. This book, my personal bias, is based on the fact that the spine supports the individual on a pure anatomic functional basis. FUNCTIONAL ANATOMY must be the "bottom line."

Any part of the person must function properly or must be considered *diseased* or *impaired*. DIS-EASE implies lack of comfort or pain. IMPAIRED means malfunctioning.

As any mechanical structure must be understood as to how it functions *normally*, so must a malfunctioning machine be studied and understood so that correction of the malfunction is *the* treatment. An abused, misused, or damaged part must be specifically located so that proper correction is possible. If this applies to machines and their function and if the human spine is a functional anatomic machine, why does this principle not apply?

It does!

The first part of this book deals with functional anatomy: how the spine is constructed and how it functions normally. It describes which tissues are capable of causing pain when they are misused or injured, *how* they are injured or misused, and the symptoms and findings leading to diagnosis. Terms are clarified. Conditions are discussed. Blame is placed where blame belongs. Labels are clarified or corrected. Decisions recommended by physicians, surgeons, and therapists are explained. In the long run, it is the patient who must make the decision and the effort. The patient's low back pain and low back impairment are at stake and are of concern.

"Oh, my aching back" must not be the lament of the industrially injured patient, the frustrated housewife, the harassed employee, or the frustrated physician. "Oh, my aching back" is a challenge that frequently can be answered and helped.

READ ON!

CHAPTER 1

What Is Low Back Pain?

Eighty percent of human beings experience low back pain at some time during their lifetimes. This statement—extrapolated from industrial statistics, medical records, and insurance figures—probably does not fully reflect the greater number of persons who have backaches that do not prevent them from working or performing activities of daily living but make their daily activities painful.

Low back pain is a common affliction whose specific cause and precise treatment are still somewhat baffling to the medical profession.

There are other diseases of the body that can and do cause low back pain. These conditions include diseases of the kidney, stomach, pancreas, and bowel; malignancies; and numerous other bone, metabolic, and systemic diseases. These disorders are always considered by the physician when low back pain is different, associated with other symptoms, or unusually persistent, or fails to respond to the recommended standard treatments.

These causes of low back pain are mentioned throughout this book, but the major concern is for the mechanical low back pain that is the most common cause of low back impairment.

WHAT IS MEANT BY MECHANICAL LOW BACK PAIN?

The spine is a mechanical structure that supports the individual from the day of birth throughout his or her life. The spine defies gravity, or at least is in balance with gravity. It supports mankind in standing and sitting and allows an individual to bend, stoop, squat, twist, turn, and, in other manners, function throughout the activities of daily living.

The normal function of the spine must be understood in order to understand abnormal function, which may cause pain and disability.

Somewhere in the tissues of the lumbar spine is a site, a spot, or a portion of those tissues that is or has been irritated, stressed, abused,

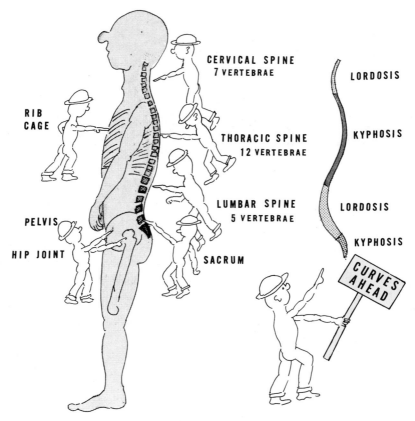

FIGURE 1. The vertebral column: the spine.

injured, used improperly, deteriorated, or even diseased. Pain can result from this tissue insult. Pain can be evaluated, understood, and remedied if the injury and the specific tissue site are clarified.

HOW DOES THE SPINE FUNCTION?

The spine is known as the vertebral column and is essentially a column of one *functional unit* upon another. These functional units, placed one upon the other and balanced upon the sacrum, keep the column erect and in good balance against gravity (Fig. 1).

The lumbar spine contains five vertebrae and forms a normal curve in the erect posture called lordosis. This lordosis is also frequently called the sway of the low back (Fig. 2). Between vertebrae are the disks, and behind the disks emerge the nerves that descend into the legs.

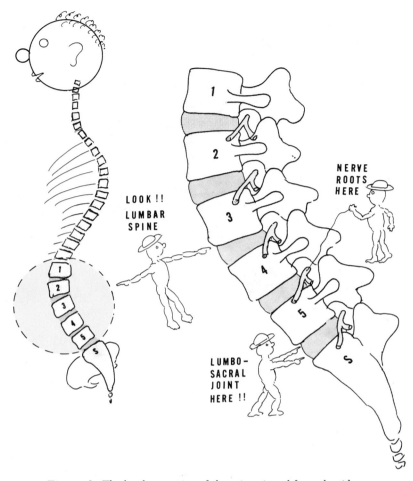

FIGURE 2. The lumbar portion of the spine viewed from the side.

The lumbar spine viewed from behind (Fig. 3) reveals the five lumbar vertebrae balanced upon the sacrum. The sacrum is contained between two broad bones of the pelvis, called *ilia*. One of the *ilia* is called an *ilium* and connects to the sacrum by the *sacroiliac joint*. Both ilia contain sockets into which the hip joints fit. These ball-and-socket joints permit movement of the ilia, and hence the pelvis and the lumbar spine.

The sacrum continues down to form the tailbone (the coccyx). The sacrum is a flat bone between the two pelvic bones (ilia) (see Fig. 3). The coccyx is formed by several small bones that resemble a tail.

The lumbar spine, with its vertebrae and their disks, is balanced upon

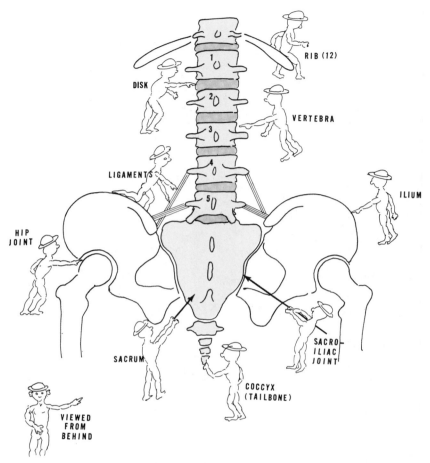

FIGURE 3. The lumbar spine viewed from behind.

the sacrum. The vertebrae form the thoracic spine upon the first lumbar vertebra.

The functional unit is the building block of the spine and therefore must be discussed in some detail. Then the entire vertebral column, in which all the functional units are placed one on top of the other, will be discussed in detail (see Fig. 2).

The Functional Unit: What Is It?

The functional unit (Fig. 4) is composed of two vertebral bodies separated by the intervertebral disk. This portion of the unit is the weight-bearing portion of the spine, which supports the body and allows bending

6

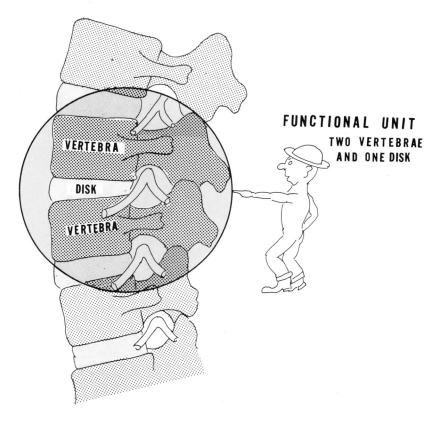

FUNCTIONAL UNIT
TWO VERTEBRAE
AND ONE DISK

VERTEBRA

DISK

VERTEBRA

FIGURE 4. Functional unit: two adjacent vertebrae with disk between.

and some turning and twisting, as in bending forward, arching backward, turning to twist, bending to sit, and arching forward in leaning, lifting, and pulling.

Each functional unit works independently *and* collectively within the vertebral column. It is, therefore, interesting and important that each functional unit be understood in order for the overall picture to become clearer.

The functional unit contains sensitive tissue that when irritated, injured, stressed, or diseased causes the patient to experience pain. The functional unit must be studied and understood in its everyday function to fully explain the cause of this pain and to indicate the tissues from which pain can occur.

The vertebral bodies (Fig. 5) are bone with a hard outer core known as the cortex and an inner bone marrow, as in other bones of the body. The marrow contains blood vessels such as arteries and veins, nerves, fat tis-

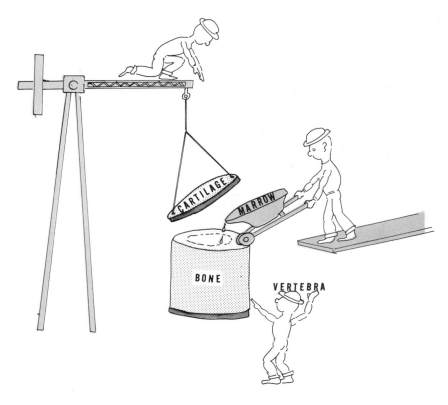

FIGURE 5. The vertebral body.

sue, and water. At each end of the vertebra, the top and the bottom, is a ring-shaped layer of cartilage. Both ends of the opposing bones are covered with cartilage, forming a joint.

Behind the vertebral bodies, there is a bony extension posteriorly (to the rear) that contains two other joints. This bony extension also forms a canal that contains the nerves of the spinal cord.

When viewed from the top (Fig. 6), the vertebral body and all the components of this bony structure can be visualized. These structures are called the pedicles, the lamina (remember this term later when back surgery is discussed), and the two rear joints: the facets. From this bony arch around the canal, the transverse processes protrude to the sides and the posterior superior spine to the rear. The back muscles and ligaments attach to these processes between any two vertebrae of a functional unit. These will be discussed in more detail later.

All components of the functional unit viewed from top down are shown in Figure 7. A side view of these structures is shown in Figure 8. It is

8

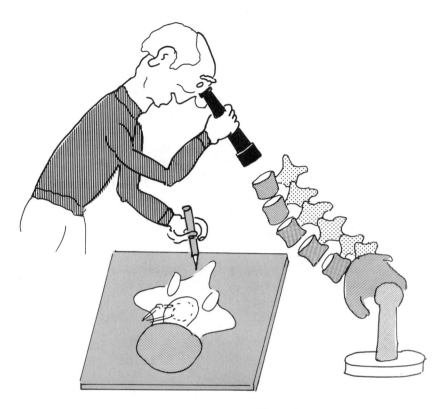

FIGURE 6. Vertebra viewed from above.

apparent from the labels "front" and "back" in Figures 7 and 8 that the functional unit is being viewed from the left side. In the front are the vertebral bodies, two of which fit one on top of the other with a disk placed between the vertebral bodies. Behind the vertebral bodies are shown the pedicles and transverse processes that form and curve around to make the spinal canal (see Fig. 7).

The muscles of the back (the erector muscles) attach to the transverse processes. The superior facets and the inferior facets form the joints behind the vertebral bodies. The vertebrae, one on top of the other, form an opening that is known as the *intervertebral foramen*. This will be shown in a later figure.

The front and the back of the spine are clearly demarcated in Figure 8, and all of the assistants are pointing to the parts contained in the functional unit: the vertebral bodies, the pedicles, the transverse processes to which attach the muscles, the facet joints, and the posterior superior spines. The joints are known as facets. The ligaments attached to the

9

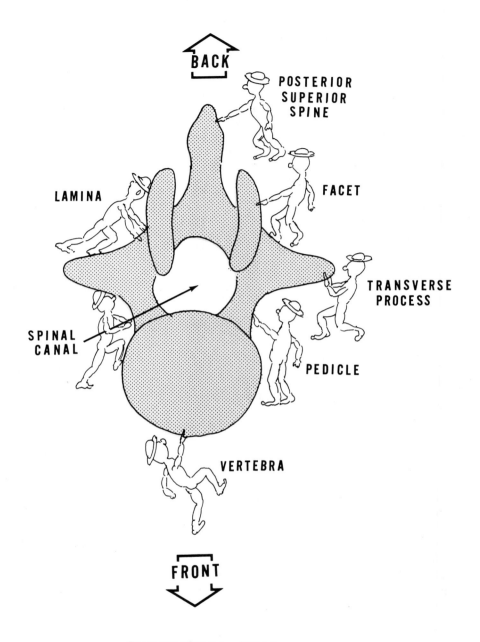

FUNCTIONAL UNIT
TOP VIEW

FIGURE 7. The functional unit viewed from the top, as shown in Figure 6.

10

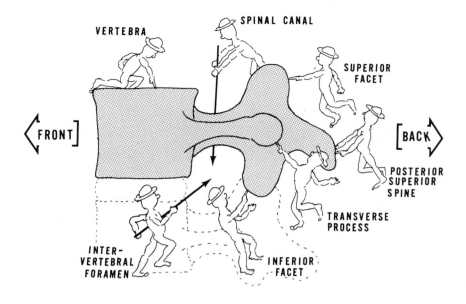

VERTEBRA

SPINAL CANAL

SUPERIOR FACET

⟨FRONT]

[BACK⟩

POSTERIOR SUPERIOR SPINE

TRANSVERSE PROCESS

INTER-VERTEBRAL FORAMEN

INFERIOR FACET

FUNCTIONAL UNIT
SIDE VIEW

FIGURE 8. Side view of the functional unit. One vertebra and the posterior structures are shown in the dark position of the drawing. The adjacent vertebra of the functional unit is shown in the dotted lines.

posterior spine and the intervertebral disk fit between the vertebrae. (see Fig. 6).

The Intervertebral Disk

The two vertebrae of each functional unit are separated by an intervertebral disk. Every pair of vertebrae of the spinal column is separated by a disk. Although there are more than 30 disks in the entire vertebral column (see Figs. 1, 2, and 3), the ones that are of concern in the low back are the five disks of the lumbar spine.

What Is a Disk?

The disk is a hydraulic system that keeps the vertebrae apart. It acts to cushion any balance or pressure and permits the functional unit to move in flexion to the front, extension to the back, and to the side (lateral flexion).

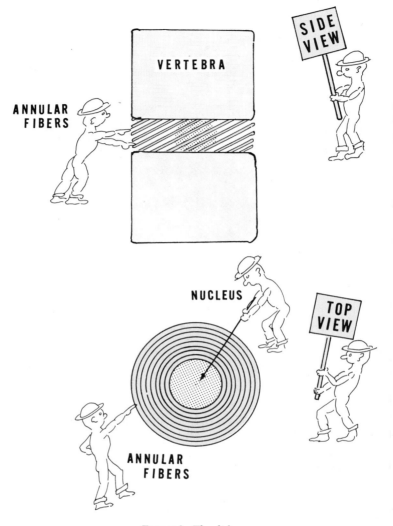

FIGURE 9. The disk.

The disk (Fig. 9) is made of two separate parts: an outer layer that is termed the annulus and a central core termed the nucleus. The disk, both the annulus and the core, contains 88 percent water. This water is held in solution within a gelatinous substance that has been called the matrix.

Throughout this gelatinous water matrix are numerous fibers that encircle the entire annulus to reinforce the disk itself. These fibers attach around the entire margin of the end cartilage plates of the vertebra and

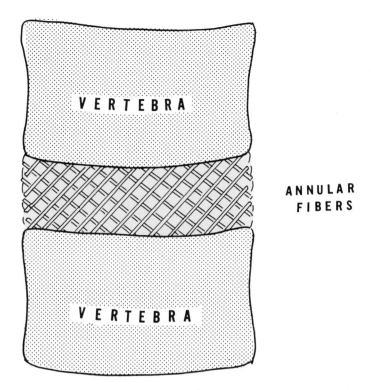

ANNULAR
FIBERS

FIGURE 10. The annular fibers of the disk.

crisscross at an angle to attach to the opposing end plates, as shown in Figure 10. Because there are many layers of annular fibers, they form a very strong reinforcement that keeps the vertebrae together and in the center completely surrounds the nucleus.

The annular fibers are layered very much as one observes in a slice of an onion. They encircle and envelop the central portion, the core of the disk known as the nucleus. When looked at as a sliced onion, but from the side view, these fibers are layered so that the first layer of fibers crosses in an oblique direction from one vertebra to the other (see Fig. 10). The next inner layer of fibers crosses from one vertebra to the other in the opposite direction, thus causing these fibers to crisscross and intertwine. Each layer of fibers goes in an opposite direction. This arrangement gives strength to the disk annulus, yet permits the vertebrae to move in any direction.

The fibers of the annulus can stretch to a limited degree; therefore, when the vertebrae are compressed together, the fibers stretch but do not tear. When the vertebrae bend on each other, the fibers can stretch

13

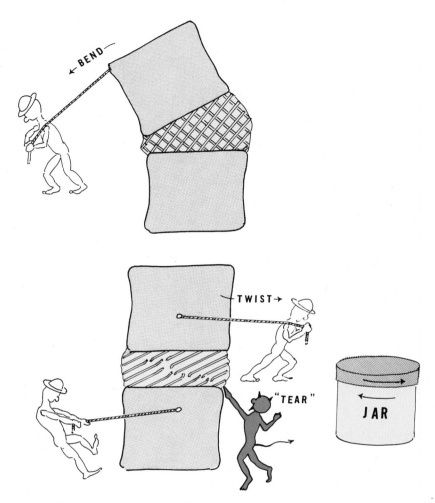

FIGURE 11. The annular fibers in the disk, allowing bending but tearing when twisted.

enough to allow bending but do not tear (Fig. 11). When the fibers are twisted, as one would picture from unscrewing the lid of a jar, the fibers become stretched more than they can allow and thus tear (Fig. 12). The outer fibers tear first and more completely than those in the layers closer to the center, the nucleus.

The annular fibers are made of tissue called collagen. Collagen is found throughout the body and is called connective tissue. It is so termed because it *connects* all the organs and tissues of the body together. Connective tissue supports organs such as the lung, stomach, liver, spleen, and

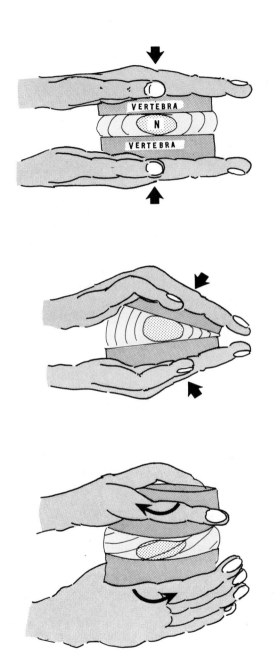

FIGURE 12. The ability of the disk to compress or bend but *not* twist.

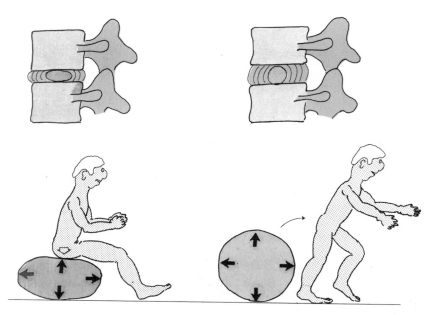

FIGURE 13. The beach ball action of the nucleus of the disk.

the bowel. It is also found in the skin, in the tissues around every joint of the body, and in the intervertebral disks of the spine.

When collagen fibers are seen through a powerful microscope, they look like springs. These springs, or collagen fibers, can stretch to the full length of the spring. When tension on the spring is released, they return to their normal size. If these springs are stretched past their point of lengthening, they tear and cannot spring back. If enough fibers of the disk annulus become torn, the nucleus, which is contained in the center of the annulus and under pressure, is no longer held in the envelope of the collagen fibers. It thus begins to leak out of its central position.

The nucleus, known as the nucleus pulposus, is found in the center of the disk. Like the rest of the disk, it is mostly water and is held within a gelatinous mass. It is held firmly within the envelope of the annulus and is centered between the end plates of the two vertebrae (see Figs. 9 and 10). The nucleus is under pressure, which keeps the vertebrae apart. It acts like an inflated beach ball on which someone sits (Fig. 13). When pressure is applied to the nucleus, the nucleus deforms, only to regain its original shape when the pressure on the nucleus is released. Thus, the disk is, in every sense of the word, a hydraulic system.

The nucleus permits the spine to bend forward and backward, always regaining its original upright position when released. Because there is a

16

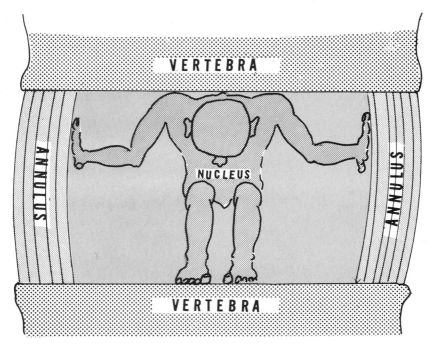

FIGURE 14. The disk nucleus: the Hercules of the spine.

disk between every one of the thirty-some vertebrae of the vertebral column, it is evident why the spine throughout its entirety can support the entire body weight, can absorb the numerous daily shocks applied to it, and can permit the spine to stoop, squat, and still regain its erect position. The spine accepts the shock of weight bearing and bending because the nucleus normally deforms and the annulus normally has elasticity (Fig. 14).

The Long Ligaments

Connecting the functional units together are long ligaments that run up and down the entire length of the spine. The ligament in the front of the spine is known as the anterior long ligament, and the ligament down the back of the vertebral bodies is known as the posterior long ligament. These long ligaments are termed *longitudinal* ligaments.

These ligaments are attached to the vertebrae in the same way a strip of tape would be applied to two building blocks stacked one upon the other (Fig. 15). They limit the amount of bending of two adjacent vertebral bodies because these ligaments do not stretch a great length. They merely

17

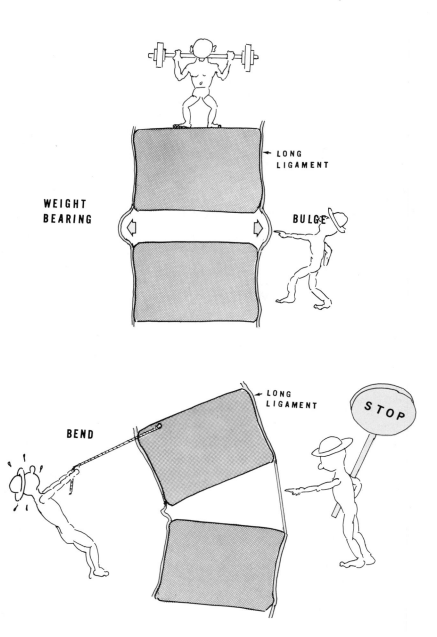

WEIGHT
BEARING

LONG
LIGAMENT

BULGE

BEND

LONG
LIGAMENT

STOP

FIGURE 15. The long ligaments of the spine.

18

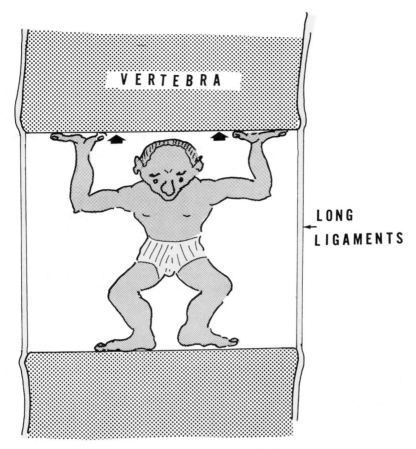

FIGURE 16. The disk pressure within makes the ligaments taut.

elongate to a specified degree, then tear or become unglued from the vertebral bodies if further stretch is imposed upon the spine.

In their passage from one vertebra to another, the long ligaments encircle the disk and form the outer layer of the intervertebral disk.

The pressure within the nucleus pushes the vertebrae apart. As the pressure of the nucleus also is directed outwardly, it causes the fibers of the long ligaments (Fig. 16) to become more taut. As the longitudinal ligaments become more taut, the spine becomes stable. If the pressure within the nucleus were to decrease, the vertebrae would come closer together and the ligaments would become slack. This approximation of the vertebrae is what happens when the disks lose some of their water from aging, disease, or injury.

19

The long ligaments contain nerves that carry sensation of pain; therefore, when they are irritated or injured in any way, pain can occur.

Neural Canal

Behind the vertebral bodies in the functional unit are bones that form a canal (see Figs. 7 and 8). Within this bony canal (a bony tube that runs the entire length of the spine from the head to the tailbone) are contained all the nerves of the spinal cord. The spinal cord, as it approaches the tail bone or the lower portion of the vertebral column, forms separate nerves that are aptly called the cauda equina. This is Latin for *horse's tail*. The cauda equina becomes separate nerves that proceed downward. The nerves of the equina individually pass through side windows of the functional unit to the hips, legs, feet, ankles, and toes. The cauda equina and the nerve roots will be discussed fully in Chapter 2.

This bony canal, viewed from top downward (see Fig. 8), has bony protrusions extending from the vertebral body on both sides, which are known as pedicles. The pedicles proceed backward from the vertebral bodies and halfway around the canal send a bony protrusion to each side, known as the transverse process. These transverse processes protrude to both sides and are a point of attachment of the muscles of the back. The back muscles will be discussed in detail later.

Proceeding posteriorly from the transverse processes, the bones enlarge to form a thickening known as lamina. From the lamina, extending upward and downward, are cartilage-covered joints known as facets (see Figs. 17 and 18).

DIRECTION OF MOVEMENT OF THE LUMBAR SPINE

The Facets: What Are They? What Do They Do?

The facets are interesting in that they are joints with surfaces that face each other, glide upon each other, and permit the spine to bend forward and backward. Because of their flat surfaces fitting into each other in a frontal plane (Fig. 17), they prevent the spine from rotating (twisting or turning) to the left or to the right to any significant degree. By their alignment, they also prevent the spine from bending sideways to any degree (Fig. 18). These facets, found uniquely in the lumbar spine, allow the lumbar spine to bend forward and backward but prevent or restrict side bending or twisting. The lumbar spine (low back) essentially can only flex or extend, that is, bend forward or backward, but can bend very little to the left or right, or twist (Fig. 19).

20

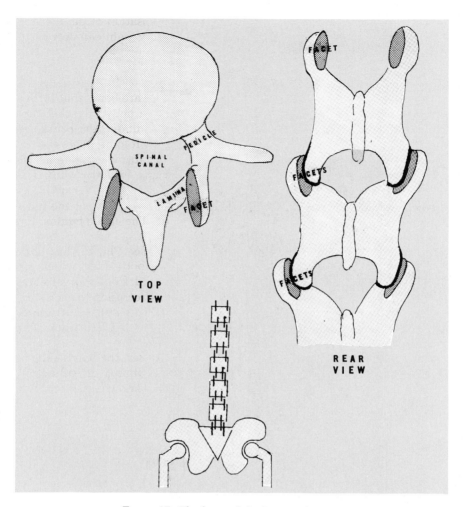

FIGURE 17. The facets of the functional unit.

Posterior Superior Spine

Proceeding posteriorly from the neural canal, the bones of the lamina, the side walls of the spinal canal, come together in the midline to form a posterior strut. This bony protrusion is known as the posterior superior spine (see Figs. 7 and 8).

21

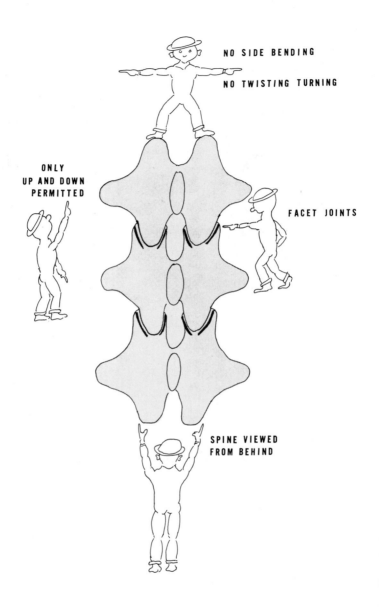

NO SIDE BENDING

NO TWISTING TURNING

ONLY
UP AND DOWN
PERMITTED

FACET JOINTS

SPINE VIEWED
FROM BEHIND

FIGURE 18. The direction of movement of the functional unit permitted and denied by the facets. Because of their alignment, the facets allow only flexion and extension but little or no side bending or twisting.

22

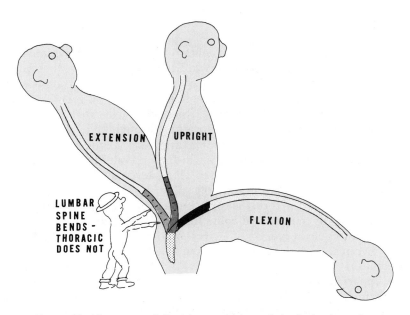

FIGURE 19. Movements of the spine: occurring *only* in the lumbar spine.

Posterior Superior Ligament

Ligaments are attached from the posterior spines of one vertebra to the next. These ligaments are known as posterior (rear) superior ligaments. They are extremely important in that as the spine bends forward, the posterior spines must separate and can do so only to the extent that the connecting (posterior superior) ligaments between two spinous processes will permit (see Fig. 12).

When the functional unit is viewed from the side as the spine bends, the vertebrae rock on each other about the nucleus. The pedicles separate, the facet joints open as they glide on each other, and the posterior superior spines separate until the ligaments intervene, stopping further flexion.

As the spine returns to the erect position, thus arching backward to regain the lordosis, the opposite occurs. The posterior ligament becomes slack. The pedicles, the facet joints, and the posterior superior spines reapproach each other. All this will be clarified when the entire lumbar spine is examined.

23

The Vertebral Column

As has been stated, the vertebral column consists of one functional unit upon the other from the sacrum upward and ultimately at the top supports the head (refer to Fig. 1). This column is not a straight structure. Rather, it is a structure with numerous curves (see Fig 1). The lower portion curves, forming the sway of the low back. Medically, this is termed lumbar lordosis. This curve occurs through five vertebrae, the lumbar vertebrae. To retain a center-of-gravity alignment, the spine above the lumbar lordosis then curves in the opposite direction, forming an opposite curve of the thoracic spine. This is termed the dorsal kyphosis. There are 12 vertebrae in the thoracic spine.

Perched on top of the thoracic spine is the neck, the cervical spine. The seven vertebrae of the cervical spine form a curve that is different from that of the thoracic curve, one that is similar to the curve of the lumbar spine: a cervical lordosis. The head is balanced on top of the entire vertebral column.

It is apparent that the vertebral column is precariously balanced upon the sacrum (Fig. 20). The sacrum is held between two broad bones that form the pelvis. The two halves of the pelvis are known as the ilia. The hip joints (Fig. 21), one on the left and one on the right, fit into the ilia through ball-bearing sockets. These ball-bearing joints permit the hip to bend, twist, turn, and extend. They simultaneously allow the pelvis to rotate about these ball-and-socket joints on each side. The pelvis essentially rotates about the hip joint.

CONTROL OF CURVATURES OF THE SPINE

Since the sacrum is firmly connected to the ilia and, in turn, supports the entire vertebral column balanced upon it, it is evident that as the sacrum tilts, so tilts the vertebral column. If the sacrum tilts forward, the lumbar spine takes a different angle and must curve backward to maintain its balance (Fig. 22). As the pelvis tilts farther, the lumbar spine increases its lordosis to regain its balance. Conversely, as the pelvis tilts in the opposite direction, the lumbar spine takes a more vertical direction: the lordosis decreases (Fig. 23).

Lumbosacral Angle

It is apparent that the degree of curvature of the spine depends on the angle of the sacrum. This is termed the lumbosacral angle (see Fig. 22).

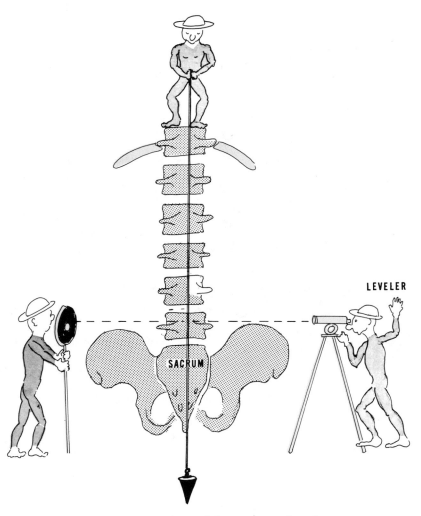

FIGURE 20. Balance of the spine upon the pelvis.

Posture

The position and the movement of the pelvis have important functions in that the pelvis maintains the body erect and influences the posture of the individual. Posture is the erect, unmoving spine.

Posture is maintained in a very efficient manner. It must be maintained

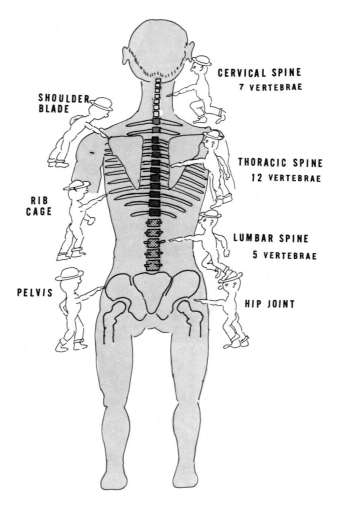

CERVICAL SPINE
7 VERTEBRAE

SHOULDER
BLADE

THORACIC SPINE
12 VERTEBRAE

RIB
CAGE

LUMBAR SPINE
5 VERTEBRAE

PELVIS

HIP JOINT

FIGURE 21. The entire vertebral column.

with very little energy expended and very little attention paid to it by the individual.

The erect spine is supported upon a reasonably flat, stable base, the sacrum. The spine, in turn, is held erect by the pressure of the disks pushing the vertebral bodies apart, causing the long ligaments to be taut. These structures maintain the erect spine. In the erect, unmoving spine, the muscles of the spine do not work, and the posterior superior ligaments are not of any significant support.

If the body sways forward, backward, or to the side to a slight degree,

26

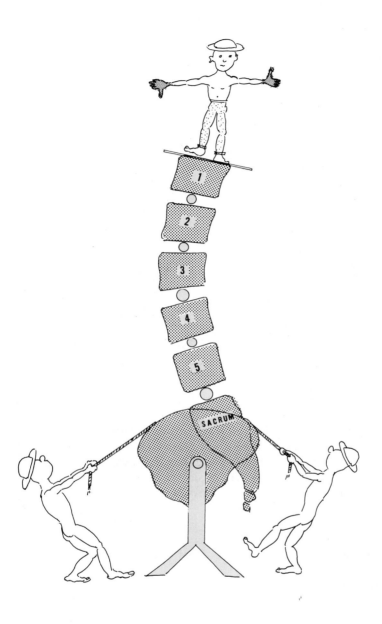

FIGURE 22. Spinal balance upon the sacrum. The lumbar spine is balanced upon the sacrum at an angle, the lumbosacral angle (see Fig. 23).

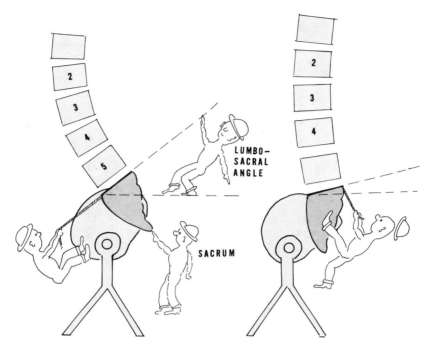

FIGURE 23. As the sacrum changes its angle, the lumbar spine curves accordingly. The direction of the sacrum is termed the lumbosacral angle. The lumbar curve is lordosis.

which the standing person does normally, the muscles are immediately notified that there is a movement away from the center of gravity. The back muscles immediately go into action, that is, they contract to prevent further bending forward, backward, or sideways. The muscles act only in brief spurts and immediately become relaxed when the spine again is erect.

The posterior and lateral ligaments are of little value in maintaining the erect posture. They are elastic enough to permit some sway movement before being called upon to prevent further sway.

Proper Posture

Proper posture has been considered to be that of a reasonably shallow lordosis on the lumbar spine. Medically, this is termed a decrease of lordosis, or flattening the sway of the back. The head, at the very top of the vertebral column, must be balanced directly above the sacrum to ensure perfect, effortless balance. This requires well-balanced curves plotted upon the center of gravity (see Fig. 1).

28

Posture is important for several reasons. Pleasing appearance of the individual demands good posture. Posture also reveals to the observer the individual's frame of mind: whether the individual is alert, rested, and energetic, or is poorly conditioned, depressed, or tired. This analysis of the patient's state of mind has been termed body language. Posture can be influenced by habit, training, and conditioning. It can also be influenced by structural changes in the shape of the vertebral bodies from disease, from injury, or from defect in the development of the spine in childhood.

Spine Balance

Viewed from the front or back, the alignment of the spine depends somewhat on the level of the pelvis. If both legs are of equal length, the pelvis should be level. The spine should then be balanced in an erect manner upon the level base (see Fig. 20).

Functional Scoliosis

A short leg upsets this pelvic balance. The pelvis drops down on the side of the short leg and is no longer level. The spine has to curve to regain balance to the center of gravity. A curve that results from a pelvis that is not level in a flexible spine is termed *functional* scoliosis. *Scoliosis* means a side-wise curvature of the spine. *Functional* implies that it is temporary without bony changes in the spine. A functional scoliosis occurs only when the person is erect and disappears when he or she is lying down.

A spinal scoliosis that is observed with a pelvis that is level may indicate that bony changes in the spine are causing the curve. This is considered a *structural* scoliosis. It does not disappear upon reclining. A scoliosis with a level pelvis, however, can be caused by unilateral muscle spasm. This functional scoliosis caused by muscle spasm will be discussed in detail in later chapters.

A pelvis that is not level, due, for instance, to a short leg, causes a functional scoliosis and has been considered to be one of the causes of low back pain, but the imbalance must exceed 1/2 inch discrepancy, that is, one pelvic brim is 1/2 inch higher than the other. This implies that, for whatever reason, the short leg is 1/2 inch or more shorter than the other leg.

Although good posture should be pain-free, poor posture may also be pain-free but is much more likely to cause pain. More information about posture as a cause of low backache will be presented when the painful spine is discussed. In this chapter, only the normal, pain-free spine is being considered.

Just as a person may stand erect with the spine well balanced over the center of gravity, the body must bend to sit and must bend forward to reach objects located ahead of the body. The spine must also be able not only to bend in a forward plane but also to do some twisting and turning. A person must not only be able to bend but also to lift. Understanding all of these functions requires full understanding of how the spine bends.

The spine bends in a well-coordinated manner. The person standing in the erect posture, as has been stated, stands erect against gravity by virtue of the pressure within the disks keeping the vertebrae apart and simultaneously placing tension upon the long ligaments. This erect spine is, in turn, supported upon a well-balanced sacral base. The ligaments other than the long ligaments (see Fig. 15) and the muscles of the spine are relaxed when the person is merely standing erect.

Muscular Control of the Bending Spine

As a person begins to bend or decides to bend forward, the body shifts slightly ahead of the center of gravity. Immediately, the sensor tissues within the back muscles send a signal to the brain that the body is off center. The muscles immediately go into action to prevent the body from bending forward too rapidly (Fig. 24). The muscles of the back that prevent the body from falling forward and ultimately allow the body to bend forward smoothly are small, very powerful, erector spinae muscles. These are the muscles of the back (Fig. 25).

The sensors of the muscles function without the person being aware of their action. They are very sensitive, spring-coiled tissues within the muscles that immediately upon being stretched send a message through the nerves to the spinal cord to the brain that stretching has occurred. The brain and spinal cord automatically and instantaneously cause the muscles of the back to react so that they do not stretch too far or too abruptly, but rather gradually and smoothly lengthen.

As the body bends farther in the forward-flexed position, as a person does when reaching down to touch the floor, each functional unit of the lumbar spine "opens up" from behind. Each unit flexes, and thus the lumbar spine flexes. (Fig. 26).

The muscles of the back that are connected to the bony portion of the functional unit must elongate to allow the functional units, and hence the lumbar spine, to flex (Fig. 27). They must do so in a smooth, gradual, controlled manner, until finally they have elongated or stretched as far as they can (see Figs. 26 and 27). The muscles of each of the five functional units of the lumbar spine elongate sufficiently to allow the separate functional units to bend. Each functional unit flexes approximately 8 to 10

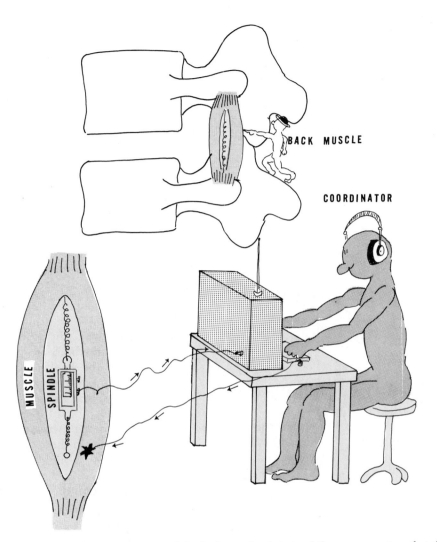

FIGURE 24. The "sensor" tissues of the back muscles that signal the nervous system that the muscle is being stretched, is lengthening, and how rapidly.

degrees (Fig. 28). Since there are five functional units in the lumbar spine, the low back flexes a total of 40 to 45 degrees. The lumbar spine bends forward approximately 45 degrees from the center of gravity (Fig. 29).

When the spine has bent 45 degrees, the muscles have stretched as far as they can, and their fibrous lining, called sheaths, now will stretch no farther. The lumbar spine is now fully bent.

31

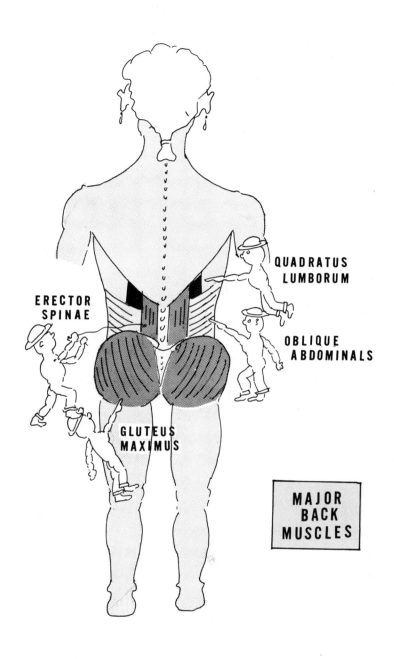

QUADRATUS
LUMBORUM

ERECTOR
SPINAE

OBLIQUE
ABDOMINALS

GLUTEUS
MAXIMUS

MAJOR
BACK
MUSCLES

FIGURE 25. The back muscles: the back extensor muscles.

32

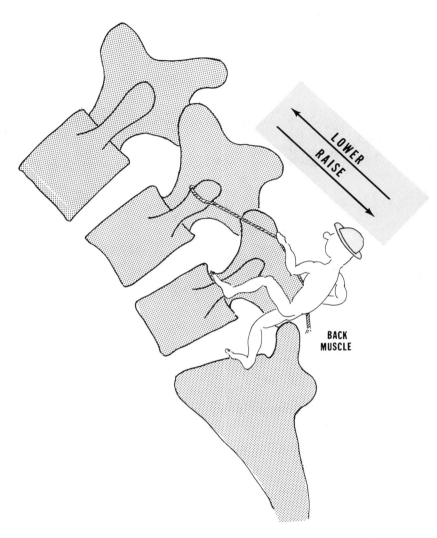

FIGURE 26. The back muscles are attached to the vertebral segments (the transverse processes), and as they lengthen, they allow the spine to bend. They essentially allow the functional unit to "open" from the rear.

Lumbar-Pelvic Rhythm: Low Back–Hip Teamwork

By the time the back muscles have elongated to their maximum, the long ligaments behind the spine—the posterior superior ligaments—have now also been stretched until they also will permit no more stretching.

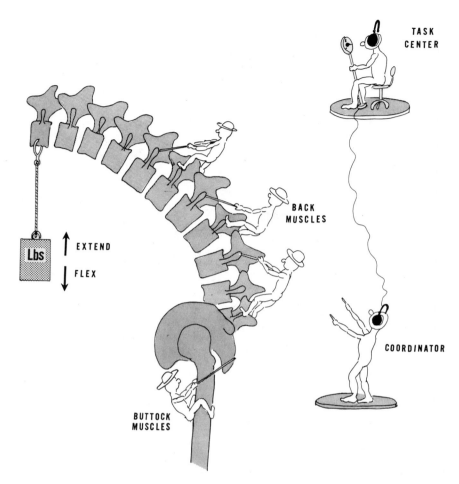

FIGURE 27. The back muscles, connecting two vertebrae each, lengthen to allow the spine to bend forward and shorten to bring the person to the upright, erect posture.

The spine will now bend no further due to the muscle sheaths and the ligaments. Any further bending of the person from this point normally occurs by further rotation of the sacrum about the hip joints.

Rotation of the pelvis and sacrum occurs by virtue of the fact that the hip and buttock muscles elongate, allowing the pelvis to bend forward symmetrically and smoothly (Fig. 30). These muscles elongate until they have been stretched to the point that their fiber sheaths will stretch no more. At that point, the buttock muscles and the posterior thigh muscles, termed the hamstrings, stop any further rotation. At this point, the entire body has bent forward to its maximum.

34

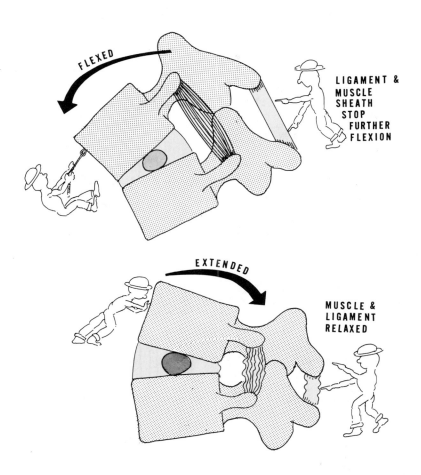

FIGURE 28. Each functional unit flexes (bends forward) as the back muscles elongate. Muscles elongate as far as their sheaths (skin) allow. Once fully stretched, the posterior ligament stops further movement. As the back arches backward, the muscles and the ligaments relax.

Good Physical Conditioning

For this smooth spine and pelvic movement to be coordinated, the muscles must be stretchable, the fibrous tissue must be elastic, and the ligaments must also be elastic. Most important, the nerve supply of the muscles that control their function must be well coordinated.

MIND OVER MATTER: MENTAL CONTROL OVER BENDING

The coordination of this muscle control of the back is under the supervision, direction, and control of the central nervous system (the brain and

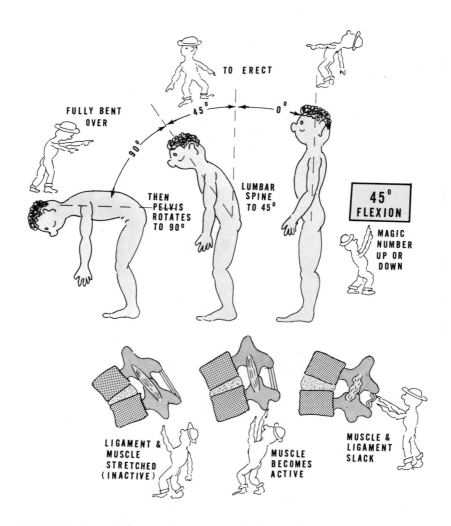

FIGURE 29. Since each functional unit opens to flex forward 8 to 10 degrees and there are five lumbar units, the lumbar spine bends forward about 45 degrees.

spinal cord). This means that the person must originate and plan the intended task in his or her mind that initiates the entire procedure of bending or lifting.

The *task itself* is the determination of how quickly, to what degree, in what direction, and how frequently bending must occur. All of these factors are determined instantaneously by the mind, usually without overt concentration on that particular object. Most tasks are done subconsciously. The object to be lifted, size of the object, the distance the object

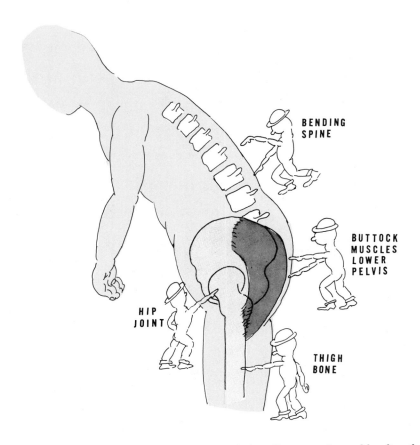

FIGURE 30. The pelvis rotates about the hip joints to allow more forward bending than the lumbar spine alone will permit.

must be lifted, and the weight of the object to be lifted are all immediately noticed by the person and fed into the mental computer to determine the exact magnitude of the intended task (Fig. 31).

How to Lift?

For example, if a heavy box is to be lifted, the direction the person must bend to pick up the box, the size of the box, and the distance from the body that it will be when it is lifted must be immediately recognized. The weight of the box must be estimated. The position of the body must be set for that particular task. The muscles are informed about the exact job to be done. The muscles must react in a coordinated manner to perform the task efficiently.

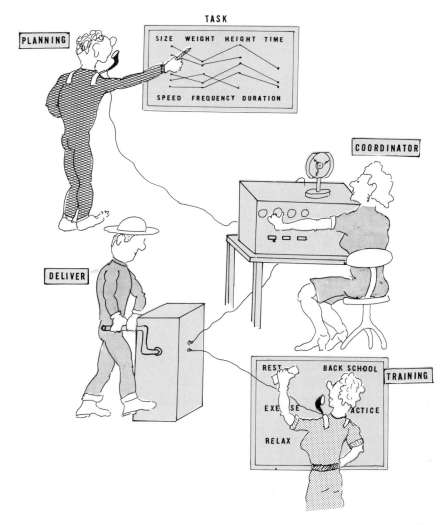

FIGURE 31. "Mental" control over the low back muscles, thus control over bending and re-straightening of the spine.

The muscles must not lift more than the size of the box. They must not lift the box abruptly or in an improper manner. If the mental computer has been well set, the task has been well organized in the person's mind, and the computer itself has been well trained by conditioning and by practice, the task is accomplished with no stress or injury, and hence *no pain*.

This sequence of events in *any* physical activity is probably the most important function of the spine that, if violated in any aspect, can cause a breakdown of the coordinated movement and impose a mechanical stress upon the back.

Once a task has been set, such as lifting the heavy box, movement of the spine and pelvis should proceed automatically. The pelvis balanced upon the legs is properly positioned to perform that job. The back bends sufficiently to reach the box. The box is lifted by the hands and arms, which immediately send information to the brain that the box has a specific size and weight. The computer automatically, instantaneously sends the required signals to the central nervous system coordinating center to accomplish that particular task.

The box is then lifted by the muscles of the back with the pelvis acting in a coordinated manner to re-extend the spine to an upright position in lifting the box. All the spinal curves that have existed in the bent-over spine are altered until the body is now fully erect. The box is now in its desired position, having been lifted with minimal effort and no duress.

Further movement of the box is again set in the mind as a new task. This new task determines the direction and position of the body and all of its muscles and ligaments that must cooperate and coordinate to achieve that task of carrying the box, changing position of the box, or putting the box down. The same muscles that did the first job are thus reoriented to perform a different task.

If the task given to the body is overwhelming because the box is heavier than the person should carry, the body will fail to accomplish its job. If the task is wrongly determined because the box is considered to be very heavy when it is actually empty, this will cause the body to make faulty effort. The body will intend lifting a heavy box that is actually light. The result will cause the body to overreact.

The converse of faulty planning can occur if the mind perceives the box to be light but the box is actually very heavy. Unless the computer of the mind corrects this error, the body will make an effort to lift a light box, only to have a heavy box become the object of lifting. The body will not be prepared for that task.

It is evident, therefore, that the task must always be correctly defined and programmed in the computer of the mind, and also be appropriate. The body must also be prepared and physically able to perform the task without any distraction. Distraction can be the result of fatigue, anger, depression, boredom, or inattention. All of these play a large part in influencing the computer of the mind. Therefore, elimination of distractions is instrumental in programming the proper task.

No matter how appropriate and well programmed the task that is presented to the computer of the mind may be, if the machinery that is set in motion is inadequate, unskilled, untrained, or poorly conditioned, the task will not be done effectively. A poorly prepared body will not be up to performing that task at that moment. Numerous examples of this will be discussed in the ensuing pages on back pain.

RETURN TO THE ERECT FROM THE BENT POSITION: LIFTING

Body flexion has been described as bending forward from the erect position to the fully bent position. This flexion is done by the lumbar spine moving from the curved, erect position to the forward, bent position in a smooth, coordinated manner.

Just as the pelvis rotates in a smooth, coordinated manner as the spine is bending forward, so must the spine now return to the erect position from the bent-over to the fully upright position. This is true whether one is lifting or merely returning to the erect posture from the bent forward position (see Fig. 29).

When the spine is fully bent forward, the pelvis is completely rotated about the hip joints. The muscles of the buttocks and posterior thigh are fully stretched at this point. The low back has fully flexed forward, with all of the muscles of the back and the ligaments fully stretched. From this flexed position, all of these movements now must be reversed to get the spine back up to a straight position.

This should be done in the following sequence:

1. The pelvis must begin rotating in the opposite direction to regain its normal erect upright angle. This rotation begins when the muscles behind the pelvis and the thighs start shortening to pull the pelvis back to the erect position. These muscles, which elongated to allow the pelvis to let the back down, must now smoothly and gradually shorten to return the pelvis to its erect position.
2. As the pelvis is rotating, the spine balanced upon the sacrum also gradually resumes its erect position. From the fully flexed position to a 45-degree forward-flexed position, the low back remains flexed and the ligaments and muscles remain stretched. Only the pelvis should rotate. The spine returns to that erect position (45 degrees of flexion) supported by the ligaments and muscle fibrous tissue. The muscles should not yet shorten.
3. The spine does not resume its normal, full erect, lordotic curve until it has reached the point of 45 degrees of flexion, which was passed on its way down in bending. The spine returns to 45 degrees of flexion because the ligaments and fibrous elements of the muscles pull the spine up, rather than because the back muscles shorten. After 45 degrees of flexion has been reached, the back muscles begin shortening.
4. At the point of regaining the erect posture with the body still bend-

ing forward 45 degrees, the pelvis has regained its derotated erect position. The spine must now regain its erect lordotic curve in the fully erect position. This is done by the muscles of the back shortening slowly and smoothly. In this phase of spinal re-extension, erector spinae muscles slowly contract. This movement brings the transverse processes, lamina, and posterior superior spines together until the normal position of the functional units of the erect spine has been reached (see Fig. 28). From 45 degrees of flexion to the fully erect position with the muscles shortening, the tension on the fibrous elements of the back muscles and the posterior superior ligaments becomes slack again. Their job has been done.

5. Once fully erect with the body well balanced over the center of gravity, the muscles and the ligaments are now relaxed. At this point, full flexion and re-extension have been accomplished.

Coordination and Conditioning Is the Key

It is apparent that a well-coordinated neuromuscular mechanism must function to properly perform the intended task. The tissues of the low back must be well conditioned, very flexible, and strong. Then, if well coordinated, the task is performed without discomfort, pain, or impairment.

Bending and Twisting

The facet joints of the lumbar spine are shaped and aligned to permit bending forward, allowing little or no bending of the spine to the side, and no twisting or turning. Forward and backward are the only directions in which the lumbar spine can bend.

A slight amount of side bending and twisting is possible when the spine has bent forward fully. This is the position of the person who has reached all the way down toward the floor. In this flexed position, the facet joints of each functional unit separate slightly. The lumbar spine can now bend sideways or twist to a greater extent than it could in the fully erect position. In the fully erect position, the facet joints are brought together, allowing no side bending or twisting movement. In forward flexion, they separate. Therefore, as a person bends down to pick up an object, the bending of the lumbar spine allows a slight amount of side bending and twisting to occur.

Acceptable Twisting While Bending

If rotation and side bending along with forward flexion are done slowly, smoothly, and gradually, these movements can be accomplished

41

without any significant discomfort. The annular fibers of the disk are stretched slightly but not enough to cause them to tear, as the facet joints prevent excessive twisting and turning.

Once fully bent forward, however, the protection that the facets afford to the disk annular fibers is decreased because the facets have moved apart to a greater degree. Separation of the facet joint permits the functional unit to twist to a greater degree than normal. This excessive twisting may tear the fibers of the annulus. Without the protection of the facet joints, all twisting stress is borne by the annular fibers. *Twisting of the disk is the only motion that can tear annular fibers* (see Fig. 11).

Straightening Up From the Bent, Twisted Position

If the body has flexed and simultaneously rotated in a *normal* manner, it must come back up the same way to regain the erect posture. This requires not only the derotation of the pelvis and the straightening of the lumbar spine, but at the same time a derotation of the rotated spine. This must be done with smooth, symmetrical, gradual movement.

If this is done carefully in a natural sequence, no problem occurs. Unfortunately, many patients bend down and simultaneously twist in picking something up from the floor that is located to one side of the body. This requires bending and twisting. During return to the erect position, if the spine does not *untwist* smoothly and symmetrically, the tissues within the functional unit can be injured and inflamed. The facet joints being "out of line" can jam, or the fibers of the disk can tear.

CHAPTER 2

Sites of Low Back Pain

Pain in the low back is the major concern of this book, but before *how* pain occurs can be discussed, we must consider *where* in the functional unit of the spine pain can occur.

Pain occurs in the back when tissues within the functional unit become irritated and cause the patient to experience pain. With the knowledge of what comprises the functional unit and how the functional unit works, we can now discuss *which* tissues within the unit are capable of causing pain and *how* these tissues are irritated. This chapter discusses conditions that cause pain and how the specific tissues capable of being painful have been irritated and misused by these movements or positions.

SITES OF TISSUE PAIN WITHIN THE FUNCTIONAL UNIT

Several types of tissue within the functional unit can cause pain when irritated. These are illustrated in Figures 32 and 33.

Is There Disk Pain?

The disk itself, always considered to be the real culprit as the main source of back pain, interestingly is *not* the major contributor to pain. The reason that the disk is not a major source of pain is that the disk is essentially a gelatinous mass of tissue with an enveloping container of collagen fibers. *There are no nerves penetrating deeply into the disk* annular fibers or into the nucleus of the disk. The nucleus of the disk is definitely insensitive and not capable of causing significant pain.

The outer layer of fibers of the envelope of the disk, the annulus, is supplied by nerves. When these outer fibers are torn, stretched, or damaged, pain can result. This means that the only portion of the disk that can cause pain is the *outer* layer of the annular fibers.

43

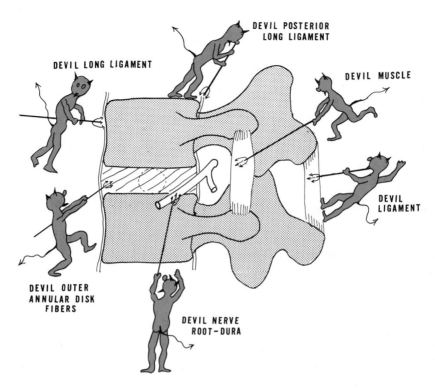

DEVIL POSTERIOR
LONG LIGAMENT

DEVIL LONG LIGAMENT

DEVIL MUSCLE

DEVIL
LIGAMENT

DEVIL OUTER
ANNULAR DISK
FIBERS

DEVIL NERVE
ROOT-DURA

FIGURE 32. Tissues within functional unit capable of causing pain when irritated. The "sensitive tissues" within the functional unit seen from the side view (left side).

The Sensitive Long Ligament

The long ligament that lines the front of the vertebral column is well supplied by nerves and will transmit pain when abused, misused, irritated, or injured in any way.

The long front and back longitudinal ligaments that protect the disk do so by forming an outer layer of the disk. They are similar to the outer layer of annular fibers. The long ligaments are considered to be a frequent source of disk pain. The front (anterior) long (longitudinal) ligament is the site of pain when irritated or damaged.

As one proceeds further from the front to back within the functional unit, the posterior longitudinal ligaments—the other long ligaments of the spine—are very sensitive. They are supplied by many nerves. Any injury, pressure, stretching, or tearing of these ligaments can cause extreme pain.

44

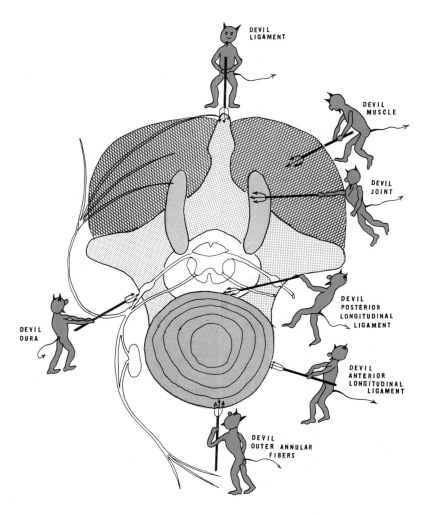

DEVIL
LIGAMENT

DEVIL
MUSCLE

DEVIL
JOINT

DEVIL
POSTERIOR
LONGITUDINAL
LIGAMENT

DEVIL
DURA

DEVIL
ANTERIOR
LONGITUDINAL
LIGAMENT

DEVIL
OUTER ANNULAR
FIBERS

FIGURE 33. Sensitive tissues within functional unit seen from top view.

SCIATIC NERVE ROOTS: A SITE OF LOW BACK AND LEG PAIN

A nerve root emerges through the foramen of each functional unit. There is a nerve root emerging between each pair of lumbar vertebrae, that is, L1–L2, L2–L3, L3–L4, L4–L5, and so forth; one nerve root emerges between lumbar 5 and the sacrum; and several nerve roots emerge through the foramen of the sacrum (Fig. 34). A small branch from each nerve root arches backward to the back muscles, to the joints, to the

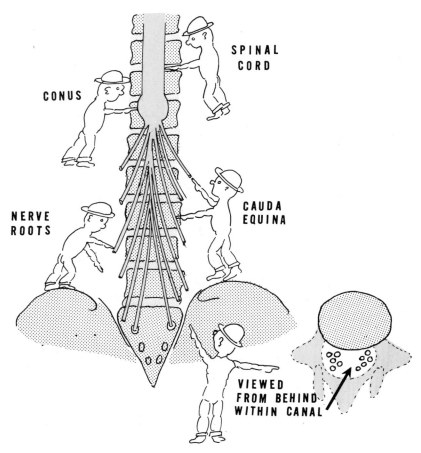

FIGURE 34. Cauda equina viewed from behind. The spinal cord descending within the spinal canal (see Fig. 7) branches out into many nerve roots as it reaches the first lumbar vertebra. These nerves resemble a horse's tail and hence are called cauda equina.

skin, and to the ligaments that carry sensation of the low back and control the back muscles. (Fig. 35).

As they emerge from the spinal canal through the intervertebral foramen, the nerve roots are contained with a dural sac. This dural sac is well supplied by nerves, making it sensitive. The dural sac is a site of pain when irritated, inflamed, or injured.

WHAT IS A NERVE ROOT?

At this point, a brief discussion of the nerves should prove helpful. The nerve roots, as they come out through the functional unit from both the

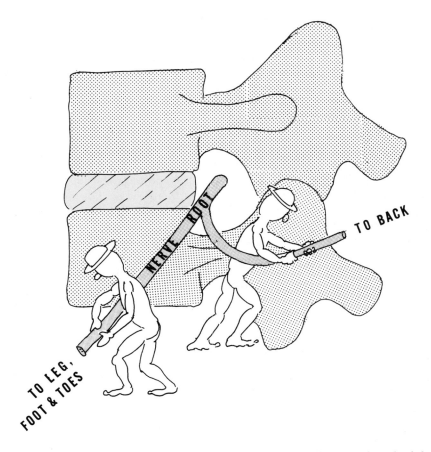

FIGURE 35. Nerve root. At each of the lumbar vertebral functional units, a branch of the cauda equina (termed a root) goes out to the specific area of the leg or foot through its specific intervertebral foramen (see Figs. 4 and 8). Each root then divides into a branch going down the leg and a branch to the low back.

left and right sides, eventually join to form the sciatic nerve. These nerves are a continuation of the spinal cord from the brain downward to eventually form branches termed the cauda equina, or horse's tail. Branches of each nerve at each functional level now become known as a *root*. A root is a combination of nerves that carry the feeling from the leg up to the cord and on to the brain. The roots also carry the nerves from the cord that control the muscles of the lower extremities.

These very fine, threadlike nerves emerge from the spinal cord at the lumbar level, and eventually join at the outer portion of the foramen to form one nerve root (see Fig. 35). This root proceeds downward into the leg after sending a small branch backward into the back muscles, joints,

47

and ligaments of the spine. The nerve roots are thus both sensory and motor in their function.

Through these nerve roots, all of the muscular functions and sensations of the legs and the back are transmitted to the spinal cord and eventually up to the brain. They convey normal sensation and the sensation of pain.

THE DURA: THE SLEEVE OF EACH ROOT

As these nerves exit through the intervertebral foramen on each side of the functional unit, they are contained within a sheath that contains spinal fluid (Fig. 36). This sheath not only protects the nerves as they come through the foramen but also gives them lubrication and a blood supply that feeds the nerves. This container, known as the dura, is an elastic tissue that is capable of stretching slightly. The dura is very resilient to significant stretching and is not subject to damage from stretching but it is a very sensitive tissue so that slight irritation from stretch of any degree can cause pain and sensitivity. The dura sheath is sensitive because it has a large nerve supply of its own.

THE WINDOW OF THE FUNCTIONAL UNIT: THE FORAMEN

The nerve itself within the sheath is well protected as it leaves the spinal canal on its way to the legs. It passes between the pedicles of the vertebrae, forming the functional unit. These adjacent pedicles form the root and floor of the foramen (Fig. 37). The front wall of the foramen is the disk with its annular fibers and its protecting posterior longitudinal ligament. The rear wall of the foramen is formed by the facet joint with its capsule, its cartilage, and its numerous small ligaments.

From our understanding of the movement of the functional units of the spine, we can see that the foramen opens as a person bends forward and closes as a person re-extends to the erect posture. In bending forward (flexing), the foramen opens. The nerve that emerges through the foramen is slightly stretched as the spine has lengthened in bending forward. As a person arches backward to resume the erect position from the bent posture, the foramen closes. As the pedicles get closer together causing the foramen to close, the nerve root in its dural container is in danger of being compressed. In re-extending to the erect posture from the bent-over posture, the spinal canal shortens as the erect posture is gained. The nerve does not get compressed in these movements because the window in a normal spine does not close sufficiently to compress the nerve and the nerve becomes slack as the spinal canal shortens. This natural protective mechanism is a beautiful example of nature's superb engineering.

The dura also becomes relaxed as the spine shortens during re-extension to the erect lordosis. The nerve can thus move away from any threatening

48

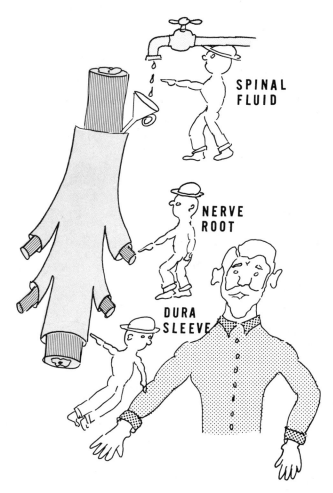

FIGURE 36. As it passes through the foramen, each nerve root is enclosed within a dura sleeve. The dura is skinlike and contains spinal fluid, small blood vessels, and small sensitive nerves.

tissue that could encroach upon the sensitive nerve and its dura. Nature has indeed assured numerous safety measures during movement of the spine.

If the nerve is damaged or irritated, the person may feel a sensation not only in the back from the branch of the nerve root that goes to the back, but also down into the leg, the foot, or ankle where the long branch of the root eventually terminates. Consequently, the nerve root at the foramen is the site of entry into the spinal cord to the brain and is also the site of the departure from the spinal cord to the lower extremities into the back. This is a very important area of the functional unit.

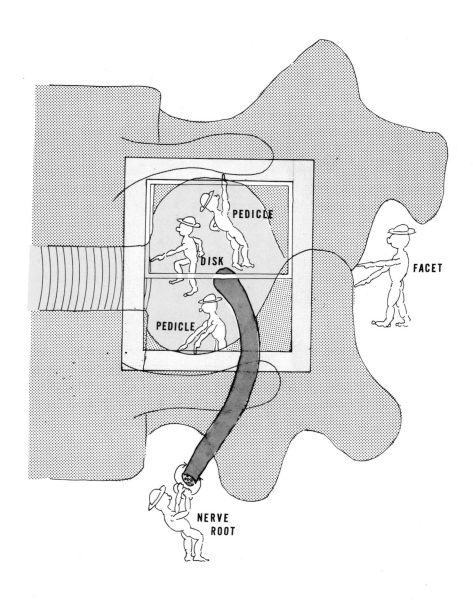

FIGURE 37. The intervertebral foramen (see Fig. 8). The "window" through which the nerve root emerges is bordered in front by the disk, above and below by the pedicles of two adjacent vertebrae, and behind by the facets.

THE FACET JOINTS OF THE SPINE

At the rear of the functional unit are the facet joints. The facet joint contains very sensitive tissues, as do most of the joints of the body (the knee, hip, foot, ankle, toe, and so forth). Facets of the spine all have tissues similar to those that make up a normal joint, namely, cartilage, capsule, joint fluid, and ligaments. The facet joint is a typical joint of the body where movement or weight bearing is required.

The facet joints are synovial joints. They are so called because they are lubricated with synovial fluid. When any synovial joint in the body becomes irritated, damaged, compressed, traumatized, or injured in any way, it may become painful and swollen. The facet joints of the functional unit may also undergo these same reactions as does any synovial joint of the body, since they are similarly constructed and contain very sensitive tissues.

THE BACK MUSCLES

As one proceeds further to the rear of the functional unit, one reaches the back muscles, known as the erector spinae muscles. These are powerful, short muscles located on each side of the spine. These muscles attach from one transverse process above to the immediate transverse process below. They combine to run the entire length of the lumbar spine.

Although these muscles are termed extensor muscles or erector spinae muscles, their function, as described in Chapter 1, is more than just extending the back. As stated, they lengthen to allow the spine to flex and shorten to retain the spine in the erect position. They shorten on one side and simultaneously lengthen on the opposite side to allow or cause side bending. They have many demands made on them (see Figs. 28 and 29).

Like muscles anywhere in the body, the erector spinae muscles are sensitive when irritated, abused, fatigued, or otherwise traumatized. They play an important part in pain production of the functional unit, and thus cause pain in the low back.

POSTERIOR SUPERIOR LONG LIGAMENT

Proceeding to the very posterior aspect of the spine, that is, toward the skin of the back, we find the long ligaments that connect the posterior superior spinous processes to each other. These ligaments are amply supplied by nerves and may cause pain if they are overstretched, damaged, or irritated in any manner (see Fig. 28).

It is apparent from this discussion that numerous tissues within the functional unit are capable of causing pain when they are misused, stretched, damaged, or otherwise irritated. The problem now is to decide *when*, *how*, and *why* these tissues can be injured, causing pain.

51

CHAPTER 3

Low Back Pain
From Poor Posture

Low back pain may be present without leg pain. Low back pain, there-fore, must of itself be discussed in the following types of patients: (1) the patient who stands in the erect posture and by that postural stance suffers low back pain; (2) the patient who bends forward and gets back pain; (3) the patient who returns to the erect position and gets back pain; and (4) the patient who suffers low backache as a result of lifting, twisting, or turning in a faulty manner.

FAULTY POSTURE CAUSING BACK PAIN

For centuries, the most common cause of postural low back pain has been considered to be an excessive *sway back*. As mankind assumed the erect position standing on both hind legs, the pelvis failed to rotate com-pletely and the lumbar spine retained a normal, physiologic curve, known as lordosis. This lordosis became known as the "sway" of the low back as it curved in above the buttocks.

As stated in the previous chapter, the angle of the sacrum within the pelvis determines the degree of angulation of the lumbar vertebrae (Fig. 38). If the lumbar spine has an excessive amount of lordosis—in other words, is excessive in its sway—back pain can result. For the sake of simplicity, the term *lordosis* will be used from here on, rather than the term *sway*.

Excessive lordosis is depicted in the pregnant woman who stands with her protruding abdomen causing her back to curve (Fig. 39). Poor posture with excessive lordosis can also result from wearing high heels (see Fig. 39). The person who stands with the low back arched and the shoul-ders "braced back" in excessive military posture may get back pain from this posture (Fig. 40).

In an activity such as ironing that requires hours of standing, the back may gradually become more arched, with resultant backache (Fig. 41).

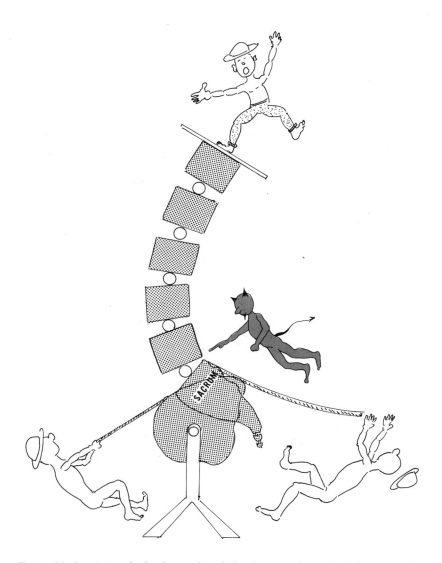

FIGURE 38. Increasing the lumbosacral angle by changing the angle of the sacrum changes the curvature of the lumbar spine. In this drawing, the lordosis is increased, possibly causing low backache.

Placing one foot up on a stool, which decreases low back lordosis, often decreases or eliminates low backache.

Faulty sleeping habits, especially lying on a soft, sagging bed or sleeping on one's stomach, cause low backache from excessive lordosis (Fig. 42). It should be noted that a soft mattress merely contours the body,

53

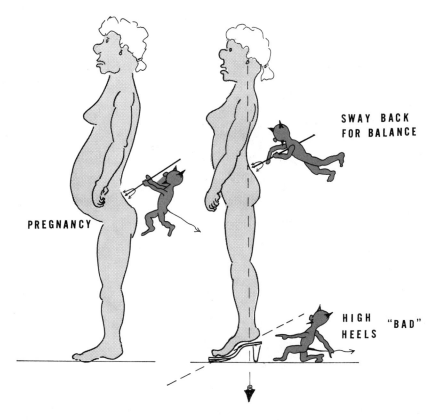

PREGNANCY

SWAY BACK
FOR BALANCE

HIGH
HEELS "BAD"

FIGURE 39. "Sway back" from pregnancy or high heels increases lordosis and can cause low backache.

whereas it is the box spring that allows a bed to sag. Thus the board under the mattress prevents the sagging, not the mattress.

Faulty sitting positions may cause low backache (Fig. 43). A chair that causes or allows excessive lordosis is undesirable. A chair with or without a pillow should assure slight flexion of the lumbar spine. A pillow should be placed at the base of the spine to ensure this posture. The height of the chair is also important. The feet should be on the floor and the thighs horizontal or even with a few degrees of hip flexion. It may be necessary to lower the chair or to place a stool under the feet.

Not all sway backs are painful. This is evidenced by the fact that everyone normally has a slight lordosis of the low back. Normal lordotic curve is to be expected. It is only when lordosis is excessive, or accentuated, that pain may result.

Proof that back pain occurs from excessive lordosis is gained by observ-

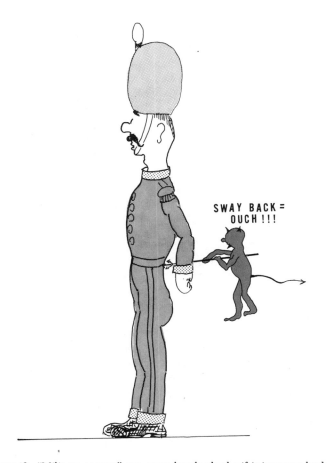

SWAY BACK =
OUCH !!!

FIGURE 40. "Military posture" can cause low backache if it increases lordosis.

ing that decreasing the sway of the back by exercise, postural training, sitting properly, standing properly, or even wearing a corset or brace that decreases lordosis also decreases low back pain.

The reason this posture creates back pain is speculative, but numerous theories have been offered to explain it. An excessive amount of lordosis of the lumbar spine causes the posterior portion of the functional unit to come closer together. The facet joints in this lordotic posture bear the entire body weight. The facet joints have been found to be sensitive and also not suitable for weight bearing. They primarily function by gliding on each other and controlling the direction of the bending and straightening lumbar spine. They also prevent lateral bending and twisting. In the lordotic, sway back posture, these joints become weight-bearing structures and can and do cause pain.

55

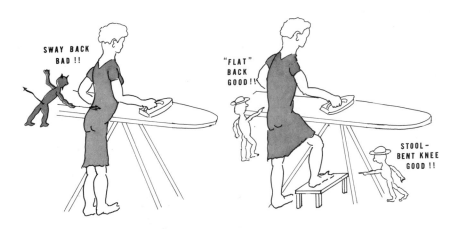

FIGURE 41. Prolonged standing with excessive lordosis plus fatigue may cause low backache. This can be eliminated by placing one foot up on a small stool.

When the back sways, the foramina also close as the pedicles approach each other. This can compress the nerves as they pass through the foramina on their way to the leg and/or to the back muscles, ligaments, and joints. Consequently, pressure upon these nerves, as well as the compression of the facets, can cause low back pain (Fig. 44).

The vertebral bodies of the functional unit, when markedly arched, squeeze the disk between the rear portions of the vertebral bodies. Since the disk is compressible and the nucleus deformable, these structures tend to deform as much as they can before bulging excessively.

How this sequence leading to low backache occurs is interesting. The anterior longitudinal ligaments stretch as far as they can in the arching process. The nucleus deforms as much as it can. The posterior long ligament becomes slack, permitting the disk to bulge backward into the spinal canal and into the foramen. Because of the sensitivity of these tissues, pressure on the posterior longitudinal ligament and the nerves as they emerge through the foramen in their dural containers results in pain.

The diagnosis of postural low back pain is the observation by the physician, therapist, nurse, or parent that the person with the back pain has an excessive lordosis. The examiner can reproduce or aggravate the back pain by further arching the patient's back. This increases the lordosis. Pain being so reproduced in the low back must be attributed to an excessive sway back. The lordotic posture may have been accentuated by poor conditioning of the patient, pregnancy, or the attempt to assume a military, erect attitude by the patient.

High heels, long the bane of the doctor's existence in causing discomforts of the feet, ankles, and knees, also contribute to low back pain. High

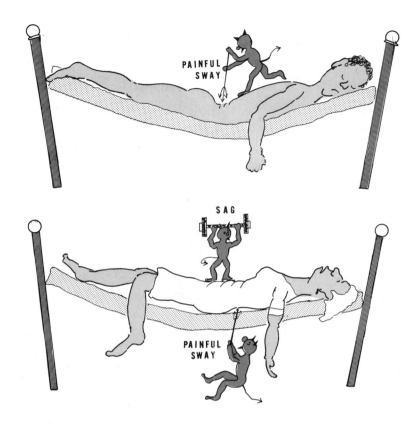

FIGURE 42. Faulty sleeping positions. Sleeping on one's stomach with a sagging mattress causes painful arching of the back **(top)**. Even lying on one's back (called supine), the soft, sagging mattress can cause low backache *(bottom)*. Obviously, the desirable bed is one with a firm mattress that does not sag because of firm under-mattress support. The objective is to prevent sag.

heels cause the body to lean forward ahead of the center of gravity, which causes the patient to arch back to regain his or her center of gravity.

The emotionally depressed patient who is tired and assumes a sad posture may well accentuate the low back lordosis. Low back pain will occur from this posture (Fig. 45).

As has been stated, the lordosis of the low back must reverse in bending forward. As the back bends forward, all of the tissues in the posterior aspect of the functional unit, including the posterior fibers of the disk annulus, are stretched. If there is rotational (twist or turning) stress exceeding the flexibility of these tissues, the disk fibers may be torn (see Figs. 11 and 12). If the tears are peripheral (outer layer) and minor, the nucleus is kept centrally and well enclosed within the inner annular fi-

57

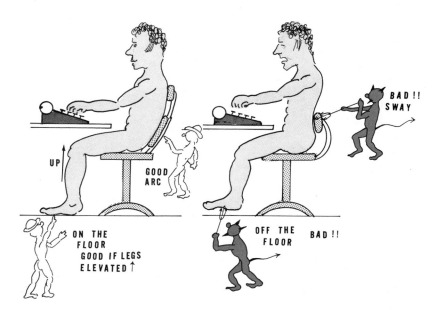

FIGURE 43. Faulty sitting posture may cause low backache. The proper low back support, feet on the floor with legs slightly elevated, table and typewriter at the right level—all must be proper to avoid low back strain.

bers. The nucleus therefore does not bulge or press forward into the spinal canal or the intervertebral foramen. There is no pressure on the nerves in their passage by the disk in the foramen; therefore, the pain is in the back with no leg symptoms.

If there has been tearing of the annulus of the disk, the annulus is weakened and becomes a potential source of further tearing. The clinical picture of the patient whose outer annular fiber has been torn is identical to that of the person who has merely bent forward and re-extended improperly with resultant pain, spasm, and scoliosis. To differentiate between merely a mechanical stress or strain and a tear in the annulus is extremely difficult.

Unfortunately, in today's medical world these low back conditions are diagnosed too frequently as a muscle spasm. Muscle spasm is given as the entire and sole cause of the back pain. However, in reviewing the entire picture, it is apparent that the muscle spasm is the end result, not the cause, or is only a contributor to the pain.

Merely to call this condition muscle spasm is as much an error as would be the diagnosis of acute appendicitis as muscle spasm of the abdominal wall. The correct diagnosis is acute appendicitis, with the abdominal wall

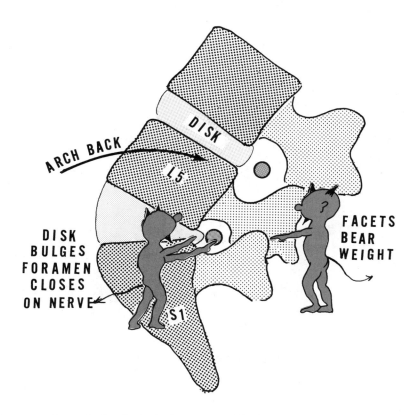

ARCH BACK

DISK

L5

DISK
BULGES
FORAMEN
CLOSES
ON NERVE

FACETS
BEAR
WEIGHT

S1

FIGURE 44. Reason for low backache from increased lordosis. By increasing the lordosis, the fifth lumbar vertebra angles back upon the sacrum. The sensitive tissues shown above become irritated, resulting in pain in the low back or down the leg.

muscle spasm merely being protective. In the low back, it is the ligamentous, muscular, disk annulus tearing or the joint stretching that has caused the muscles to go into spasm. The *strain* has been the movement that has caused the problem, but the *sprain* has been the tissue reaction to this insult. Spasm is merely protective initially but ultimately becomes a contributor to the back pain.

If the annular fibers are torn sufficiently to permit the nucleus to bulge, the resulting back pain persists longer. If the nucleus is permitted to bulge to one side into the intervertebral foramina rather than straight posteriorly, the nerves to the legs may be compressed, and leg pain as well as back pain may occur.

Back pain with spasm and scoliosis combined with simultaneous leg pain will be discussed in a subsequent chapter. Tearing of the annular

59

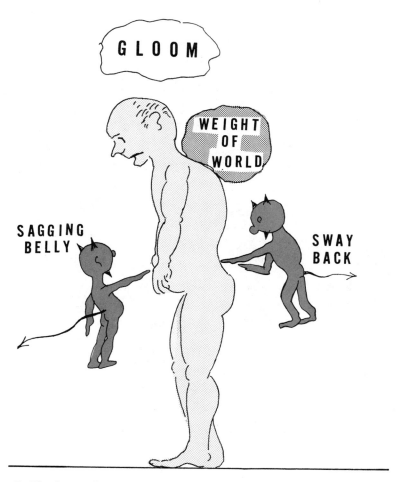

FIGURE 45. The depressed posture causing low back pain. Not only the posture but the depression make the patient more prone to having backache.

fibers in the central portion of the disk causes bulging to compress the posterior long ligament. This long ligament is exquisitely sensitive and itself may cause the muscles to go into spasm, which causes further pain and limitation of flexion.

This prolongation of pain and spasm, usually brief in a simple sprain, implies a more serious degree of back pain when it is due to the fact that annular fibers have torn and the disk has been permitted to bulge. This central bulge due to annular tear merely makes the condition more prolonged and resistant to treatment and predisposes to ultimate recurrences.

In this condition, the clinical story told to the examiner is important, as is the requirement that the examination to depict this particular occurrence be performed properly. No special test, be it x-ray, electromyography, examination, or other procedures, will be of marked assistance. Therefore, the diagnosis is made by careful history taking, precise examination, and symptoms persisting longer in spite of proper treatment.

It is apparent, therefore, that low back pain occurs from faulty use; for example, improper bending, improper re-extending from the bent position to the erect position, and improper lifting all will cause back pain. Just as prevention is important, treatment of the acute condition is also important. The pain, its prevention, and its treatment will be discussed in the chapters that follow.

CHAPTER 4

Low Back Pain From
Improper Bending and Lifting

As described in previous chapters, a person can stand erect with the muscles and ligaments of the back completely relaxed. Erect posture is maintained by the pressure within the disks that keeps the vertebrae apart, causing the long ligaments of the functional unit to be taut. As soon as the person bends forward, moving slightly ahead of the center of gravity, the muscles of the back contract immediately to prevent rapid bending forward. From there on, as the person continues to bend, the muscles of the back slowly elongate to allow the back to flex. Once the body has bent forward 45 degrees from the erect posture, the lumbar spine no longer can bend. From there on, the pelvis rotates to allow the body to bend farther down.

Not only must the muscles of the back be well coordinated to allow the spine to bend 45 degrees forward, but the muscles of the pelvis must also elongate for simultaneous rotation of the pelvis. The tissues of the back, the pelvis, and posterior thigh muscles must also be sufficiently flexible to allow this forward bending.

THE DECONDITIONED INDIVIDUAL

In an extremely deconditioned person, the tissues of the back and legs do not stretch and elongate to the length necessary to permit complete, pain-free flexion. Therefore, as this deconditioned person bends forward, all the sensitive tissues that normally should lengthen (such as the back muscles and back ligaments) do not fully extend; pain can result.

For example, if one leads a sedentary life from Monday through Friday and on Saturday does an excessive amount of work, such as gardening, exercising, or lifting, that requires stretching, one may experience low back pain. If a physician or therapist examines this person, the examination will reveal that as this person attempts to bend, the tissues of the back do not stretch adequately. The normal reversal of the lumbar spine from

62

its normal erect lordosis to the forward bent position does not occur.

If the back has been held in a lordotic posture for many days, weeks, months, or even years—such as a secretary using the wrong type of chair—the low back muscles and other tissues may shorten into this posture. The tissues of the lordotic back will tend to shorten and remain shortened. This shortening of tissues is known as fibrous contracture, which is a thickening of the tissues, causing them to lose their elasticity. Now, when the patient attempts to bend forward, these tissues do not elongate because of their inflexibility. This may cause back pain in the patient who now attempts to bend forward only to be restricted by the tightened tissues that have resulted from prolonged, persistent lordotic curve. This condition, considered to be a cause of back pain, can usually be diagnosed by observation and examination.

As the back normally bends only to approximately 45 degrees of forward flexion, the remainder of the bending forward must occur at the pelvis. To allow the pelvis to rotate, the muscles behind the thighs and in the buttocks must also be flexible. The long muscles behind the thigh, so-called hamstring muscles, must elongate to allow pelvis rotation. If the hamstring muscles are excessively tight, the pelvis is prevented from rotating long before it has accomplished its full expected movement. The remainder of bending becomes imposed upon the low back, the lumbar spine. As the lumbar spine can bend only approximately 8 to 10 degrees at each functional unit if the pelvis is stopped midway in forward rotation, each functional unit must then bend excessively. The tissues of the low back now must exceed the 8 to 10 degrees of normal flexion. Becoming overstretched causes low back pain. The person who exhibits this type of low back pain gives a history that is self-evident. The patient claims excessive activity after prolonged inactivity or poor conditioning. This situation usually is not serious and is self-limited; with rest, gradual reconditioning, and simple flexibility exercises, the patient makes a good recovery.

The back, however, may be restricted in its flexibility not by poor conditioning, but by the mental status of the individual. The person who is emotionally uptight, cannot relax, and is tense becomes tense in all of the tissues of the body, including the neck, arm, and chest. All of these tissues that have been made tense by emotional tension also restrict the amount of flexibility of the low back, and the same situation occurs in bending forward as occurs in a person who bends forward and has limitation due to poor flexibility. The end results are the same: LOW BACK PAIN.

The physician or therapist examines the individual as he or she bends forward. The low back does not achieve the normal reversal of the lordosis and the pelvis does not simultaneously rotate. To the trained observer, this is evident; to the patient, it may be felt but not observed.

BACK PAIN FROM REGAINING THE ERECT POSITION:
STRAIGHTENING UP THE WRONG WAY

Once a person has fully flexed and is bent forward at the lumbar spine with the pelvis rotated and the low back lordosis reversed, the person has now bent sufficiently so that the fingers may approach the ground in front of the individual. The person now must regain the erect position. To do this, the pelvis must derotate first with the spine remaining flexed. This continues until the entire body is 45 degrees ahead of the center of gravity. Then, and only then, should the lumbar spine gradually begin to regain its lordosis until the full erect posture has been reached. The muscles of the back of the lumbar spine do not shorten or contract until the spine has regained 45 degrees of forward flexion. The back muscles then gradually and slowly shorten. They do so in a smooth, controlled manner until the full erect position of the spine upon the derotated pelvis has been reached (Fig. 46).

This sequence of movement may be violated when a person regains the lordotic curve of the back before the pelvis is completely rotated so that the low back regains the lordosis in a forward-bent position. The upper portion of the body remains ahead of the center of gravity, causing the muscles to work excessively with mechanical inefficiency. The conditions that are known to cause lordotic back pain are now present, but this time there is additional aggravation in that the body is ahead of the center of gravity, imposing more mechanical demand upon the back muscles (Fig. 47).

There are several reasons why a person may bend forward and improperly regain the erect posture.

1. The person may be untrained and therefore unskilled.
2. The person may be well trained but at the moment of bending and regaining the erect position, or lifting, is distracted due to anger, fatigue, or depression (Fig. 48).
3. The person miscalculates the lifting task and therefore lifts in an erratic manner. An example of this is the person who sets the desired task, such as lifting a 10-lb bag, only to find that the bag weighs 50 lb. The effort is not adequate for the task (Fig. 49). The converse may be true in that the person attempts to lift a 50-lb bag with this intention, only to find that the object lifted weighs 10 lb. Here the effort overshoots the mark, and the patient responds with distress.

If a person is injured in a faulty re-extension from the bent position due to any of the above three causes, the following conditions occur in the functional units, causing pain. The back muscles are made to contract

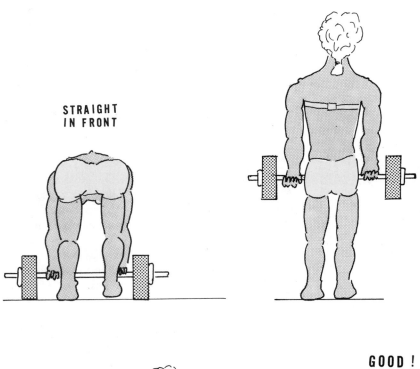

STRAIGHT
IN FRONT

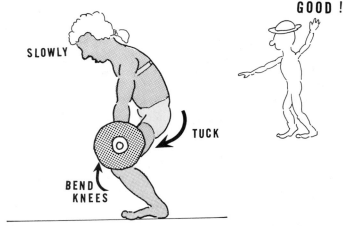

SLOWLY

TUCK

BEND
KNEES

GOOD !

FIGURE 46. Proper bending and lifting.

65

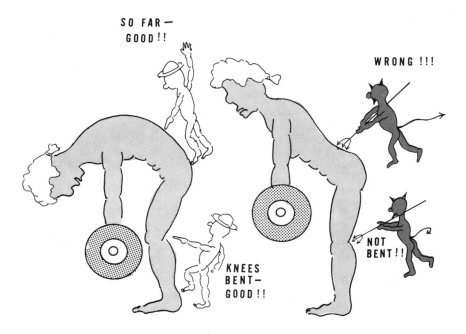

FIGURE 47. Improper bending and lifting. Regaining the low back lordosis too soon in lifting and with the knees not bent causes low back pain.

excessively and shorten abruptly. They become inflamed and painful. These muscles may go into spasm because they have been injured, inflamed, or abused. Spasm is actually a sustained muscular contraction that does not relax.

If the spasm occurs bilaterally, that is, on both sides of the spine, the spine remains erect; however, when the person attempts to bend forward, the muscles do not relax sufficiently to allow the spine to bend forward. The person then not only is unable to bend forward but walks and stands with a "rigid" spine. Any attempt at movement requiring these contracted muscles to relax is extremely difficult and painful.

Because the muscles are in spasm, the entire spinal balance is upset. Merely standing or sitting erect is done in a faulty manner because the muscles and ligaments that should be relaxed to allow proper standing and sitting posture remain shortened.

Should the muscles on only one side of the spine become irritated and in spasm, the spine becomes pulled to one side. When visualized from behind, the person is twisted to the left or to the right depending on which side of the back muscles are in spasm.

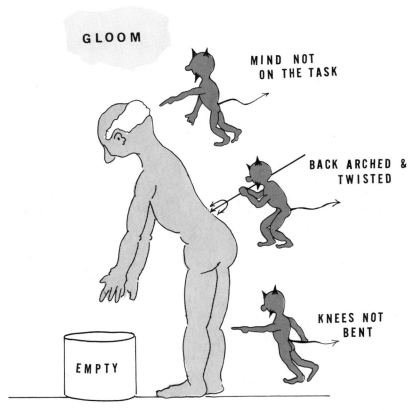

GLOOM

MIND NOT
ON THE TASK

BACK ARCHED &
TWISTED

KNEES NOT
BENT

EMPTY

FIGURE 48. Distraction that causes faulty bending and lifting, causing low back pain.

This twisting of the spine to one side is known as *acute scoliosis*. Scoliosis is abnormal lateral curving of the spine. The patient in spasm presents to the examiner in a rigid manner: unable to bend forward, twisted to one side, with the twist becoming more accentuated on any attempt to bend forward further. This person is unable to function, unable to bend, and unable to sit comfortably. If examined at this time, the muscles are tender and firm and may even be in nodules. This mechanical low back pain and disability have resulted from having bent forward then returned to the erect posture in a faulty manner (Fig. 50).

PAIN FROM TWISTING OF THE SPINE IN LIFTING

A person who has bent forward and regained the erect posture in a faulty manner and also has bent forward and turned to either the left or

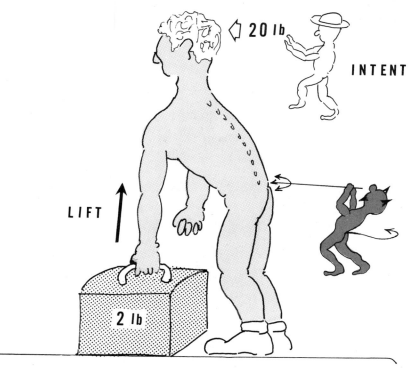

FIGURE 49. Miscalculation of lifting effort. If the person intends to lift an object considered to weigh 20 lb that weighs only 2 lb, the person *overlifts* and thus can injure the back. The opposite, an *intended* lift of 2 lb that is actually 20 lb, can equally cause a low back *underlift* injury.

right side may now compound the back problem. In this condition, the back may or may not regain its lordosis too soon in getting back to the erect position but *does not return from the rotated position* in the proper manner. This person does not derotate properly. The spine has not moved properly, thus injuring or straining tissues that cause pain (Fig. 51).

The person who has bent forward and at the same time rotated in bending down to pick up an object that is to one side of the body rather than in front of the body may "throw the back out" if the erect posture is improperly regained. If the person has returned to the erect position without proper simultaneous derotation, the back has been strained and goes into one-sided spasm. He or she now stands or walks slightly bent forward and twisted to one side. Standing fully erect becomes impossible. Bending forward is limited, as is bending to the side. The patient now has what can be termed an *acute lumbosacral strain* and *sprain* with *resultant muscle spasm* (see Fig. 36, Scoliosis).

68

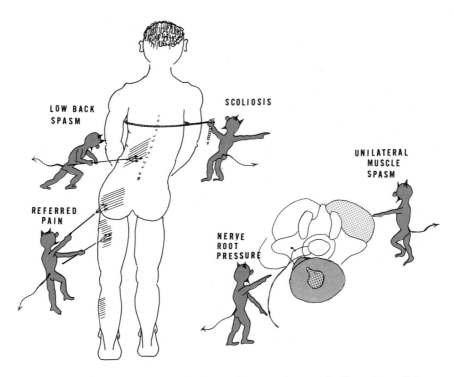

FIGURE 50. Acute scoliosis: due to low back muscle spasm. On one side (shown in small figure to right), the back is pulled (twisted) to one side of midline. This is called functional scoliosis. Spine becomes straight when spasm ceases.

The mechanism of pain production in this condition is irritation of the tissues that were discussed as pain producing in previous chapters. These are as follows:

1. The ligaments have been excessively stretched and become painful.
2. The muscles are or have been abused, reacting with spasm. They may have been irritated from having been overstretched.
3. The joints of the facets have been brought together abruptly as the spine has been re-extended and, being "off center" from the twisted position, become "jammed" and thus inflamed.
4. The foramina of the functional unit that were opened in the forward-flexed position have closed asymmetrically as the spine re-extends.
5. The nerves in their passage through the foramina now become compressed on the side to which the spine bent. The foramina are nar-

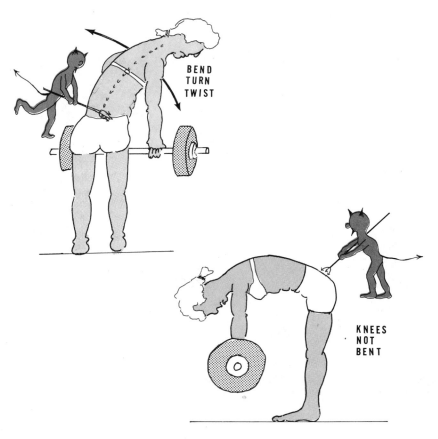

FIGURE 51. Faulty bending over and returning to erect in a "twisting" manner can cause low back strain if done with legs straight, and not returning from bent-over posture to erect by slowly and correctly *un*twisting.

rowed on the bent (concave) side as compared with the opposite side.

A good example of this type of abnormal painful lifting maneuver is the person who bends forward to lift a suitcase that is to one side of midline and must be picked up by bending forward and twisting to one side. As the person comes back up, lifting the briefcase or the suitcase without gradually resuming the forward-facing position, he or she returns to the erect position improperly and the back becomes jammed, causing acute pain.

70

If the person has twisted sufficiently far in bending forward and to one side, not only the joints, the muscles, and the ligaments become involved, but the fibers of the disk annulus may also be torn. The annular fibers of the disk, as has been stated, permit flexion and extension but do not permit excessive rotation or twisting, or they may actually tear. Since the annular fibers in the periphery of the disk are sensitive, pain may result when they are torn.

There is no specific test known to medical science that determines the fact that annular fibers have been torn rather then merely ligaments, muscles, and joints being involved. There is no evidence of the tearing of the annular fibers on x-ray films. This diagnosis is made merely from the examination and the history.

The normal spine and its function have now been fully evaluated. We can turn to the next chapter and discuss how pain can occur when the spine is abused, misused, or damaged in any way.

CHAPTER 5

Low Back Pain
From Unusual Activities

Low back pain resulting from spinal column stress can occur from activities as innocuous as sneezing, stepping down steps that are not present, stepping into a hole, coming up unexpectedly under an overhead beam, and numerous other examples. Such activities put mechanical stress upon the spine that at the moment of the stress may be in an awkward position, such as bending, twisting, and arching.

The common sneeze is a good example of this. A person sneezes without being aware that the sneeze is about to occur. Consequently, this person may sneeze while in the awkward position of standing erect, bending over, twisted to one side. The sneeze causes the muscles of the abdomen and the back to contract violently. A cough can do the same thing. These muscle contractions can catch the back unprepared and result in pain (Fig. 52).

A person may be descending stairs expecting each stair to be approximately 12 inches in height, but one of the stairs is either missing or of a different height. As this person steps down to the missing step—steps a distance of 24 inches—this jars the back, usually with an abrupt hyperextension. Pain can result (Fig. 53).

A person may be sitting on a chair that breaks and causes the person to fall backward suddenly. Low back pain can result. These are examples that are momentary and catch the back unprepared with violent muscular contraction, as well as imposing an acute mechanical compression force upon the lumbar spine.

THE TENSE PERSON

The person who is nervous, tense, uptight, fatigued, or depressed very frequently can make movements and actions that catch the body unprepared. If repeated episodes of this occur, the back can be weakened and can become more susceptible to subsequent minor injuries. When these

72

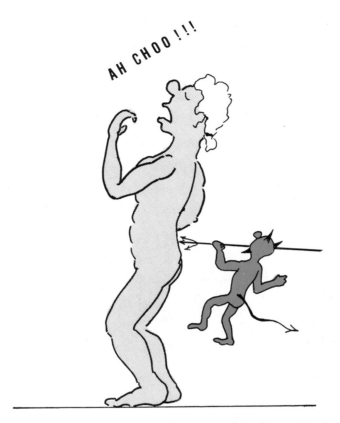

FIGURE 52. A sneeze may "catch the back unprepared for the stress" and cause low back strain.

activities occur, the powerful muscles of the back act in a very small distance with a great deal of powerful contraction. They literally jam the joints together; these joints have been specified as being sensitive, and thus inflammation results from this injury.

WHAT IS INFLAMMATION?

Inflammation is a medical term that is not to be confused with infection. There is no bug, no bacteria, no agent that causes this inflammation. Inflammation is merely the reaction of the tissues that have been abused.

Inflammation is microscopic damage to tissues. There is immediate swelling as fluid accumulates around these injured tissues. There is simultaneous microscopic bleeding as the small blood vessels, known as capil-

73

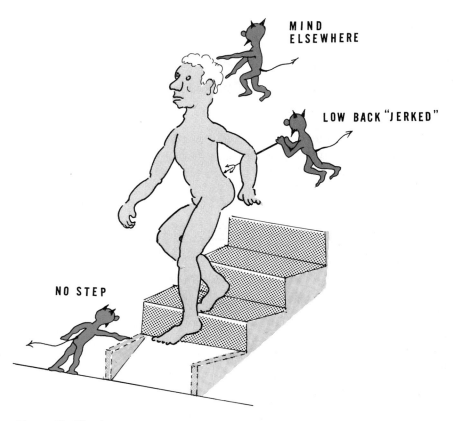

MIND ELSEWHERE

LOW BACK "JERKED"

NO STEP

FIGURE 53. The absent step. Stepping down upon a step that is not there can jar the back. This is another example of the mind being upon a "task" and the wrong, unexpected task being performed, resulting in a low back strain/sprain. This back injury can occur from stepping into an unseen hole, stepping off a curb of unexpected height, and other similar situations.

laries, ooze tissue fluids, which causes edema. There may actually be slight hemorrhage, which is not visible on the outer surface of the skin and thus is not visible to the patient or the examiner. When these tissues are irritated by inflammation, the muscles around them immediately go into protective spasm.

SPASM: IS IT PROTECTIVE?

Protective spasm is nature's attempt to prevent a part moving or being moved because of tissues having been damaged. Consequently, until the damaged tissues lose their inflammation, the muscles very frequently may remain in spasm.

74

The protective spasm unwittingly becomes a source of more inflammation and more pain. The spasm does so by squeezing the damaged tissues, causing more fluid to accumulate. More important, the spasm by preventing movement keeps the fluid that has been formed there from being removed by the normal body mechanisms. A vicious cycle has thus been set up. Trauma, injury, stress of tissues, microscopic tearing, edema, fluid, even microscopic hemorrhage, protective spasm—the cycle goes on with pain and eventually limitation. These damaged tissues cause a limitation of movement. This limitation is caused not only by the muscles going into spasm, but by their inability to relax after they go into spasm.

As was stated in the first chapter, the back muscles must gradually relax, elongate, and stretch to allow the back to bend. They also must shorten slowly, gradually, and smoothly to make the back return to the erect position. If the back has been irritated, the frequent tissue sites that have been enumerated in Chapter 1 become inflamed. The muscles go into spasm to prevent those parts from moving until healing occurs. As the patient now attempts to bend, twist, turn, or even sit, these muscles do not elongate (relax). The low back therefore becomes more painful and restricted in movement. Pain leads to impairment, and impairment may lead to disability.

If these inflamed tissues are to be properly treated, the condition must be recognized and the exact phase of this vicious cycle identified, as follows:

1. At first, pain occurs from the inflammation of the tissues.
2. Secondary pain occurs from the protective spasm.
3. This in turn causes a tertiary increase of the inflammation.

The goal of treatment after a proper examination is to break this cycle. Treatment will be discussed in detail in a subsequent chapter, but suffice it to say that proper understanding of all these conditions is vital not only for the patient, but for the therapist, the doctor, or the nurse who enters the picture of the injured low back.

It is apparent, therefore, that low back pain may occur from faulty use, such as improper bending; improper re-extending from the bent position to the erect position; improper lifting; a sudden, unexpected twist; a certain jerk from a misstep; stepping into a hole; or sneezing. All may cause back pain. Both prevention and treatment of the acute condition are important and will be discussed in subsequent chapters. The pain must be clarified so as to relieve the symptoms but also to prevent recurrence.

CHAPTER 6

Low Back Pain With Leg Pain: The Ruptured Disk

If the disk bulges, ruptures, slips, or herniates, whatever term is used, the nucleus either ruptures out of its annular container or pushes the remaining untorn annular fibers out into the spinal canal or into the intervertebral foramen.

There are numerous terms describing this occurrence, and all may gain acceptance. It is the concept that is important and the understanding of what is happening that matters. As was stated in early chapters, the nucleus is under a great deal of pressure, held between the opposing end plates of the vertebrae and surrounded by annular fibers. If the fibers tear, the pressure within the nucleus exerts force in an attempt for the nucleus to escape. It cannot escape through the end plates, so it forces its way outward to the periphery. (Fig. 54).

If the nucleus reaches the contents of the spinal canal or of the intervertebral foramen, there are pressure and irritation of the tissues contained therein, and pain and disability result.

Because the posterior longitudinal ligament lines the front of the spinal canal, is essentially the outer layer of the annulus, and is sensitive, *low back pain can result*. Within the intervertebral foramen lie the nerve roots that have two branches—one branch to the low back and the larger branch down the leg to various aspects of the leg, foot, ankle, and toes. Pain results from pressure on these tissues and is felt in the area to which the irritated nerves go.

Leg pain that accompanies and is considered to be related to low back injury can be pain in either leg felt in the front of the thigh, the back part of the thigh, or below the knee into the calf or ankle area.

The exact distribution of this plan described by the patient is of great value in helping the doctor during the examination to determine where, to what degree, and at which level (functional unit) in the lumbar spine the nerve has been irritated (Fig. 55).

76

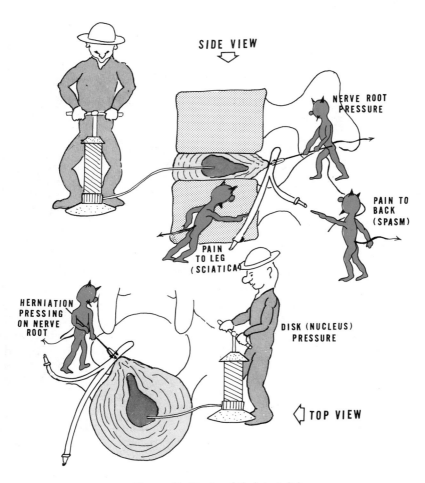

FIGURE 54. Ruptured (bulging) disk.

SCIATICA

A patient may have leg pain originating from the lumbar spine without back pain or may have both back pain and leg pain. Leg pain existing and originating from the back is medically termed *sciatica* (Fig. 56).

WHAT IS ROOT PAIN?

Sciatica, which is sciatic nerve pain, is considered to result from irritation or inflammation of the nerve roots. The nerve roots emerging from

77

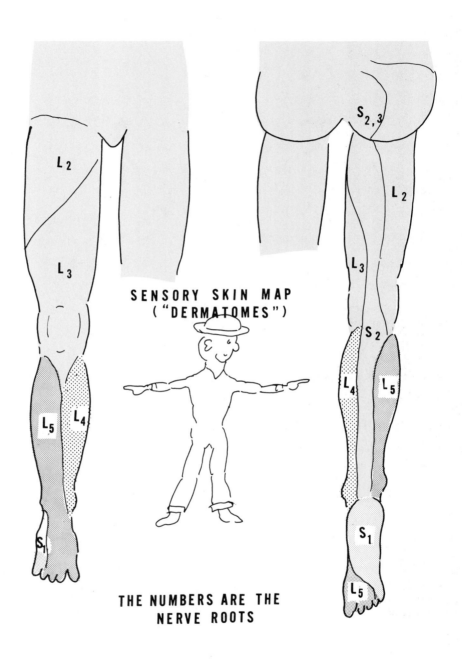

SENSORY SKIN MAP
("DERMATOMES")

THE NUMBERS ARE THE
NERVE ROOTS

FIGURE 55. The skin area of the leg is supplied by a specific nerve root. The patient points to where in the leg the pain or numbness is noted. The examiner can similarly note the specific root.

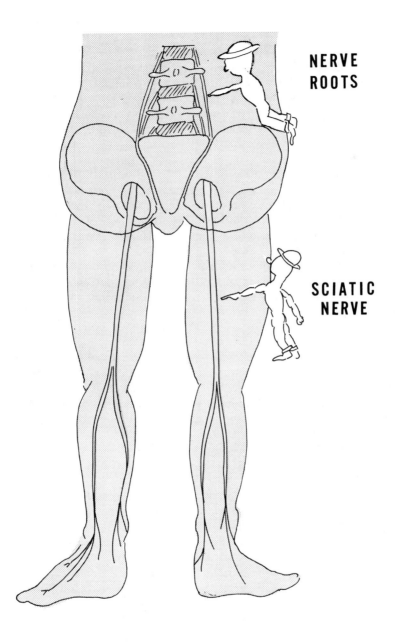

NERVE ROOTS

SCIATIC NERVE

FIGURE 56. Many roots emerging from the lumbar spine foramina regroup to form a large common nerve: the sciatic, which descends behind the leg to rebranch into nerves to various muscles and "dermatomes" (see Fig. 55).

the foramina are also known as radicles; therefore, radicular pain is pain that the patient feels radiating from the back into its ultimate distribution into the legs.

In radiculitis, which is defined as inflammation of the radicle or the nerve root, it is the nerve root that is irritated. The patient feels symptoms in and along the course of that nerve in the leg.

This pain can be described in numerous ways. It can be nagging, aching, stabbing, shooting, or a burning sensation felt in the leg in the distribution of the specific nerve root.

DERMATOMES: THE SKIN MAP OF NERVES

The distribution of nerve roots in the leg is fairly specific. The pain may be felt in the area of the buttocks, in the rear of the thigh, in the outside skin area of the thigh, as far as the knee, or even below the knee into the ankles and toes (see Fig. 55).

The patient may volunteer information describing the sensation of pain or discomfort into the region of the thigh, leg, or foot, or the doctor may have to elicit this from the patient by asking questions.

MECHANISM OF PAIN

Frequently, the pain is felt only with certain movements or in certain positions that the patient assumes. It is important that these positions be carefully noted so that the mechanism by which the nerves are irritated can be fully understood. The history elicited from the patient will determine if these movements have been the initial cause of or are directly responsible for nerve root irritation.

ROOTS OF THE SCIATIC NERVE

Two nerve roots principally make up the sciatic nerve (Fig. 57). These are termed the fifth lumbar and the first sacral roots, and they are the nerve roots that radiate down the back portion of the thigh, the buttocks, the outer portion of the thigh, the calf, the ankle, and the toes.

The fifth lumbar (L_5) nerve leaves the spine through the foramen between the fourth and fifth lumbar vertebrae. The first sacral (S_1) nerve root leaves below the fifth vertebra, in the space between it and the first sacral vertebra, or the sacrum (Fig. 57). These foramina can be reviewed by referring to the pictures of the spine in the first chapter (see Figs. 34 and 35).

These nerve roots, as shown in Figure 35, have two branches, one going down the leg and the other branching back into the muscles of the back.

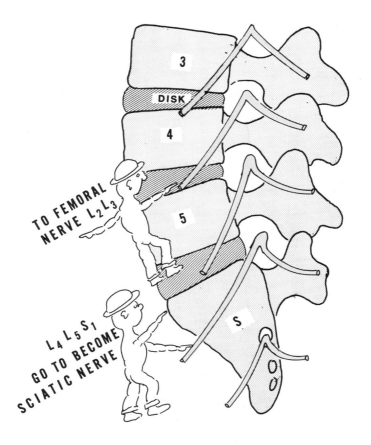

FIGURE 57. Sciatic nerve roots. The fourth and fifth lumbar nerves and the sacral nerve form the sciatic nerve. This nerve goes down the back of the leg to the foot and toes. The second and third lumbar nerves do *not* go into the sciatic nerve. They merge to form the femoral nerve, which goes down the *front* of the thigh to the thigh muscles.

Therefore, irritation of these nerves can cause pain down the leg and pain and spasm of the back muscles.

These nerves are both motor and sensory in their function. The nerve roots that are motor go to specific muscles of the leg. The S_1 root goes to the calf muscles, which allow the person to rise up on the toes. The L_5 root goes to the muscle of the front of the lower leg (the anterior tibialis muscle) that picks up the foot at the ankle. This muscle allows the foot to clear the floor when one walks and allows the person to walk on the heels. The muscle controlled by L_5 also picks up the big toe (extensor hallucis longus), as shown in Figure 58. The L_3–L_4 nerves go to the thigh muscles.

81

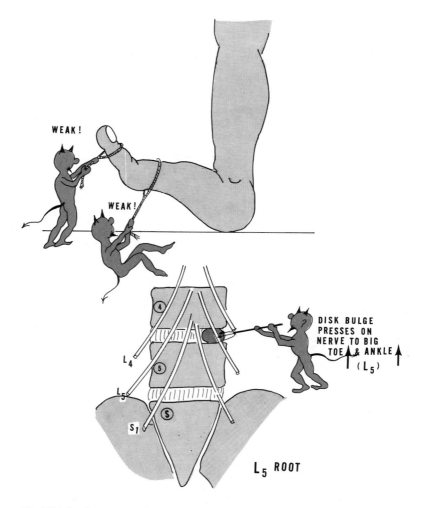

FIGURE 58. Fifth lumbar nerve. The fifth lumbar nerve root descends leg to furnish the muscles that "pick up" the foot and the big toes. If a disk (or tumor or arthritic spur) damages this nerve, the patient drags the foot.

These thigh muscles extend (straighten) the knee and permit a person to do a bend at the knees, do a deep knee bend, rise from a sitting position, climb or descend stairs, and do squats. These nerves permit the patient to walk, run, jump, and so forth by virtue of the fact that they control the muscles that perform these activities.

These nerve roots also have a sensory function in that they carry sensation from tissues of the leg and of the back. They carry the sensation of touch, of feeling, and of hot or cold, and they also, unfortunately, carry sensations of pain. Irritation of the nerve roots, therefore, can cause pain by mere irritation of the sensory portion of the nerves, or it can cause numbness of the particular portion of the leg that receives its nerve supply from that particular root. The sensation of numbness may be merely a lack of feeling or may be described by the patient as tingling, aching, or burning.

NERVE PRESSURE

Acute pressure or traction on a nerve root can cause pain without numbness. Acute or brief irritation of a nerve root can cause an unusual sensation described by the patient as tingling, aching, or burning. Often, more prolonged pressure or traction or more severe irritation will result in numbness. Therefore, numbness replacing pain in the distribution of the nerve does not indicate improvement but may indicate more ominous nerve irritation.

Numbness is claimed by the patient who can describe the sensation and designate the region of the leg where that sensation is felt. The physician confirms the specific area of numbness by stroking the leg with a finger, pin, or cotton rubbed along the skin. This determines if the skin is sensitive throughout all of these areas.

Each specific area of the skin of the legs is controlled and supplied by a particular nerve root. These very specific areas therefore can be claimed as sites of pain or numbness by the patient and confirmed by the doctor's examination as areas of impaired sensation to either light touch or to pinprick (see Fig. 55). They are frequently called the areas of root irritation.

Compromise of the motor portion of the nerve root can lead to weakness or to paralysis of the muscles served by the specific nerve roots. The patient may complain of weakness but usually will describe the weakness as a particular loss of function. The patient may claim that the foot drags, cannot run, cannot rise up on the toes, or limps. The nerve root causing the weakness in turn causes that impaired function, and in this way localizes the specific nerve root involved.

REFLEXES: THE DEEP TENDON JERKS

Muscles function by virtue of being connected to a bone by a tendon. This muscle-tendon unit pulls upon the bone, causing it to move at the joint. A muscle bends the knee joint by attaching to the two bones that form the knee joint. A muscle and its tendon attach to the bone of the lower leg to straighten the knee. A muscle and its tendon attach from the lower leg to the heel of the foot to move the foot in the direction required to get up on the toes.

Each muscle that is connected to a tendon has a specific nerve supplying it. Each tendon also therefore relates to a specific nerve. Striking or hitting a tendon, as the physician does with a rubber hammer, acutely stretches that tendon. The response to that acute tendon stretch is for the muscle to abruptly shorten. This reaction constitutes a tendon reflex (Fig. 59). Tendon reflexes thus demonstrate that the muscle is capable of reacting when stretched. This implies that the muscle has a functioning nerve supply.

The tendon of the thigh muscle that attaches to the lower leg below the kneecap elicits a reflex known as the knee jerk. This is the reflex response of hitting the tendon below the kneecap. The knee jerk tests the front thigh muscles and their nerve roots L_3–L_4.

The tendon behind the lower leg at the ankle is responsible for the ankle jerk. This is the Achilles tendon of the calf muscles, which are served by the S_1 nerve root. Loss of this reflex indicates that the S_1 nerve root is not functioning.

The knee jerk (K.J.) and ankle jerk (A.J.) reflexes are routinely tested to determine the integrity of nerve roots L_3–L_4 and S_1. There is *no* reflex to test L_5, as the muscles innervated by this root have *no* specific tendon.

Where the patient feels pain or numbness is, therefore, of definite value in indicating where in the spine injury or inflammation has occurred. Strength, lack of strength, or fatigue of a muscle implicates a specific nerve root.

The ability to go up and down on one's toes is a function of the calf muscle, which in turn is the function of the S_1 nerve root. The ability to pick one's toes up and clear the floor while walking so one does not scuff one's foot in walking is a function of L_5. The knee jerk tests L_2, and the ankle jerk tests the S_1 nerve root. They are inadvertently or intentionally complained about by the patient, who may or may not realize that this pain, loss of sensation, or loss of motor control comes from the low back by virtue of specific nerve roots being involved.

LASEGUE TEST: THE STRAIGHT LEG RAISING (S.L.R.) TEST

One of the painful conditions that patients frequently complain of and doctors test for is a sciatica caused by the stretching of the sciatic nerve. This painful reaction, the S.L.R., occurs because the sciatic nerve behind the thigh going into the lower leg cannot be stretched without causing pain because it is irritated. The nerve is stretched by flexing the leg at the hip with the knee straight (Fig. 60).

Normally, in this movement, the sciatic nerve has enough flexibility to stretch without pain. If the nerve is irritated or is abnormally stretched, it cannot be stretched farther without causing pain. Bending the leg at the hip with the knee straight elicits pain when the nerve is irritated. This test

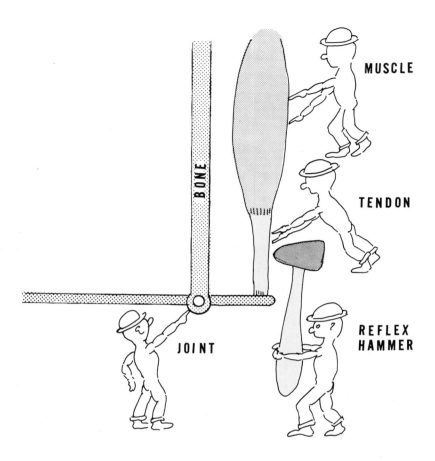

FIGURE 59. Tendon reflex. Tapping a tendon, as in this picture with a reflex hammer, causes the muscle to contract ("jerk") if its nerve supply is intact.

indicating nerve irritation is termed a positive straight leg raising test or S.L.R. This test was initially described by a French physician Lasegue and now bears his name. A positive Lasegue test occurs if pain results from raising the straight leg.

The sciatic nerve is stretched when a person stands and bends down to touch the floor without bending the knee. In this movement, the hip is also bent, stretching the sciatic nerve roots. This is why patients who have sciatica have pain down the leg on attempting to bend forward to touch the floor, to pick up objects. They have pain when lying and raising the leg up straight, or when sitting and straightening the knee in a horizontal direction (see Fig. 60). All of these are sciatic nerve stretch pain tests.

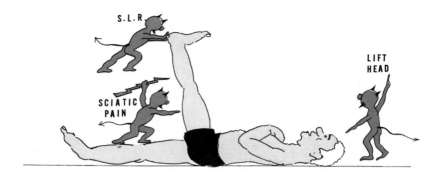

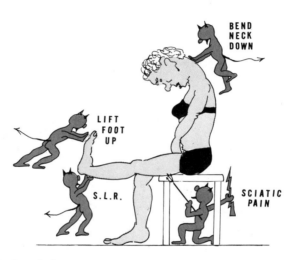

FIGURE 60. Straight leg raising test (S.L.R.) is done lying or sitting. If pain is caused by lifting the straight leg and further aggravated by placing chin on the chest, the sciatic nerve roots are irritated.

Positive S.L.R. Test

A doctor reporting a positive straight leg raising test indicates that the nerve that is being stretched on straight leg raising is inflamed, or resistant to being stretched.

BACK SPASM WITH SCIATICA

Nature always responds to a painful inflamed tissue and prevents it from being irritated. Therefore, the muscles of the legs will go into spasm to prevent the leg from being elevated, or bent at the hip. The back muscles will go into spasm to prevent the back from bending, which also

86

stretches the nerve. The picture of the patient with sciatica becomes quite clear.

SCIATIC SCOLIOSIS

In this condition, the back does not bend (Fig. 61). It may also be twisted to one side as the nerve roots that are irritated come out of either the left or the right side (see Fig. 50). The leg does not bend forward at the hip and therefore does not permit the patient to bend down when the leg is straight. The mechanism of sciatica becomes apparent.

Irritation, compression, or inflammation of a nerve root can occur anywhere along the distribution of that nerve, from the spinal cord from which it begins, through the intervertebral foramen where it leaves the spinal canal, or in the distribution in the leg from the buttocks to the ankles and toes. The major decision of the doctor in examining a patient with this complaint is to determine where and why the nerve is irritated, from what tissues, and what must be done to eliminate or decrease the pain in order to prevent further loss of function of that particular nerve.

In the patient with sciatic type of pain, unless the root branch that goes from the foramen to the back tissues is markedly involved, the back pain need not develop, merely leg pain. The leg pain indicates irritation of the long branch of the nerve root (see Fig. 57). If both branches, the one down the leg and the one to the back, are equally inflamed along their course, the patient can and will experience back pain and leg pain.

FEMORAL NERVE RADICULITIS

More nerves than just L_5 and S_1 leave the spinal canal to go down into the patient's legs. The nerves above L_5 are designated L_4, L_3, and L_2. They also leave the spinal column and go down the leg (see Fig. 57). However, they have a different course down the leg. Medically, this is known as nerve root distribution. These nerves (L_2, L_3, and L_4) do not go down the back of the leg into the calf, but rather go down the front of the leg to the muscles of the knee and the thigh.

By virtue of their specific distribution, if these nerves are irritated, they will cause weakness of the thigh muscles. This weakness will make it difficult for the patient to do a deep knee bend, go up and down stairs, or get in and out of a chair.

The reflex defect will not be the lack of the ankle jerk response to the doctor's reflex hammer. In this case, the knee jerk will be diminished. The reflex is elicited by tapping the tendon in front of the leg below the knee cap.

The skin sensation of these nerves is not in the buttocks, the back of the thigh, or the calf. There is primarily some degree of pain, sensation, or

87

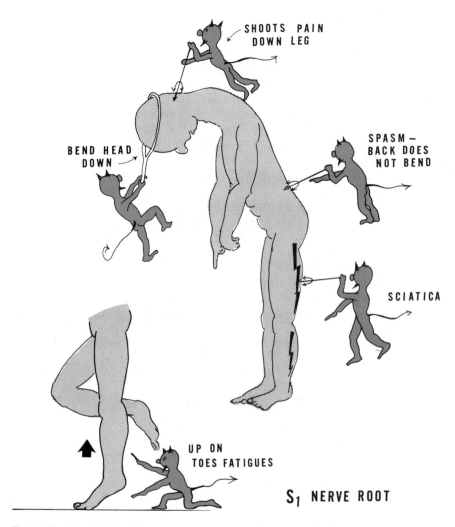

SHOOTS PAIN
DOWN LEG

BEND HEAD
DOWN →

SPASM –
BACK DOES
NOT BEND

SCIATICA

UP ON
TOES FATIGUES

S₁ NERVE ROOT

FIGURE 61. Limited flexibility and pain pattern in a ruptured disk. The low back is "rigid," does not bend, and is straight. There is pain in leg in attempting to bend forward, aggravated by bending neck. If the S_1 root is involved, there may be difficulty getting up and down on the toes.

numbness in the front part of the thigh and the knee region (see Fig. 55).

These nerves do not stretch when the leg is straight, so straight leg raising test for these nerves is not considered abnormal. With these nerves irritated, a stretch pain test similar to the straight leg raising test (S.L.R.) to the lower nerve roots is possible. As the nerve passes down the front of the leg, the patient is tested in the prone position (Fig. 62). In this posi-

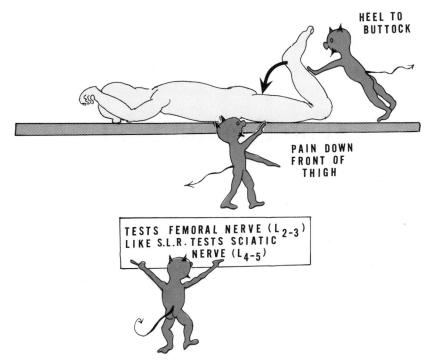

HEEL TO
BUTTOCK

PAIN DOWN
FRONT OF
THIGH

TESTS FEMORAL NERVE (L$_{2-3}$)
LIKE S.L.R. TESTS SCIATIC
NERVE (L$_{4-5}$)

FIGURE 62. Femoral nerve stretch test.

tion of lying on the stomach and the leg extended at the hip, the heel is brought toward the buttocks. Whereas with the *normal* (unaffected) leg the heel of that foot will approach the buttocks without pain, on the affected side the knee will be limited in its flexion and pain will be felt in front of the thigh.

ACUTE SCOLIOSIS DUE TO NERVE ROOT PRESSURE

Regardless of the level of nerve root irritation (L$_5$ or S$_1$ with positive S.L.R. or L$_3$-L$_4$ with positive femoral nerve stretch pain), the roots that go to the back may be irritated and cause muscle spasm. This is true of a herniated lumbar disk or any condition that irritates the nerve root as it passes through the foramen. The resultant spasm of the back muscles will prevent the back from flexing (bending over). If the spasm is one-sided, a scoliosis will occur (see Fig. 50).

Numerous tests can be performed if the pain sensations, numbness, and weakness persist or fail to respond to treatment. These tests are performed to determine *what* is causing the pressure upon the nerve. These tests will also clarify *where:* at which functional unit level the pressure exists.

89

CHAPTER 7

The Examination

The *history* is a term used medically to imply a disclosure by the patient to the physician of the events related to the problem. The problem here is low back pain.

The disclosure is usually a sequence of events volunteered by the patient. This is often directed by the physician so that all pertinent factors are disclosed. Without direction, the patient may not make certain disclosures, because he or she does not consider them important or related. Yet these same disclosures may be very important to the physician.

A question-and-answer session frequently occurs between patient and physician or between patient's relative (spouse or parent) and the physician.

WHAT IS IMPORTANT?

Site of pain indicates the tissue area of the spine that is involved. The site may be indicated by the patient pointing to or giving a verbal description of the site. The low back may be all that is specified, but *where* in the back must be further clarified. The site may be precisely designated at the lumbosacral area. It may be across the entire low back. The site of pain may be in the back spine or higher toward the rib cage. Words the patient uses—such as "my hips," "my kidneys," or "my disk"—are, per se, nonspecific but require further clarification by the questions of the physician.

HOW DID PAIN BEGIN?

Onset of pain indicates the action that initially caused the pain and ultimately may denote the *position or movement that caused, causes, or aggravates the pain*. Through knowledge of the mechanics of the lumbosacral spine, the movement of the spine causing pain can be indicated. For instance, *standing*, which causes weight bearing with the normal lumbar lordosis, may relieve the pain incurred by sitting or bending. Sitting flexes the lumbar spine and, thus, stretches the back muscles and back ligaments. These are known to be sensitive tissues that, when stretched, cause pain. The history, volunteered or answered by careful questioning, reveals the specific movements or postures causing pain.

Onset of pain can be determined by the following questions. Was the pain brought on by merely bending over or by lifting? Was the object lifted heavy, bulky, or awkward? Was the object picked up directly in front of the person or to the side, causing the back to twist or turn? Did the person slip while lifting? Was the person aware of the magnitude of the object to be lifted, its size, weight, and how high to lift and place it?

Was the person tired, bored, angry, impatient, or depressed *at the time of lifting or bending?* To reveal that the person was any of these at the time of the examination is not significant, but that this condition did exist *at the time of lifting* or bending *is* significant.

Was the action that initiated the injury a single effort or one of many repetitions that could have caused fatigue, boredom, or temporary distraction?

All of these and many other similar examples can be stated. This is known as *present illness:* the history of the current complaint.

DESCRIBE THE PAIN

All sensations have a quality, a description, or a characteristic. Pain is a subjective sensation that may indicate to the physician from which tissue the pain possibly occurs. An ache may be muscular or ligamentous. Burning may involve fascia or nerve. Soreness is often muscular. Stinging may be ligamentous. Tingling may be a nerve sensation, as is shooting pain. No single term necessarily applies to one specific tissue in every patient, but these terms indicate the direction for further studies.

Intensity of pain. How severe? This is a qualitative measure of pain that only the patient can determine. Mild or severe? Bearable, nagging, or excruciating? Intolerable or numb? These terms may indicate the severity of the injury to the tissue or indicate the tolerance of the patient to the pain.

Recent studies of chronic pain by experts in this field have designated the psychological value of specific terms applied to pain sensation. Use of certain terms alerts the knowledgeable physician as to the patient's frame of mind and the psychological meaning of the pain claimed by the patient. These are terms such as devastating, killing, overwhelming, intolerable, ravaging, demoralizing, and so forth. A family physician who knows the patient and has the confidence of the patient is always better able to evaluate the psychological status of the person giving the history.

WHERE IS THE PAIN?

The person suffering pain may point to the site of pain, indicate the location of the pain, or even indicate an organ where the pain is considered to originate: "in my low back," "in my hip," "in my buttocks," "in my sciatic nerve." All these terms are frequently used and indicate to the physician the general tissue area to be investigated.

Many physicians ask a patient to draw the area or site of pain. Front and back drawings of a person permit a patient to note by Xs, shading, lines, circles, or other means where the pain is felt. These drawings assist the examiner who knows correct anatomy and precise nerve pathways to determine exact tissues involved or to suspect exaggeration, imagination, or even deception on the part of the patient.

WHEN IS THE PAIN?

The answer to this question may be one of the most informative aspects of the history. The movement(s) or position(s) that causes the pain describes the precise spinal movement and which tissue of the functional unit is irritated. To refresh the reader's memory, the functional unit is two vertebrae, the disk, and the numerous tissues contained therein from which pain can.occur. This has been thoroughly described and illustrated in the early chapters and can be reviewed profitably.

Postural pain is noted after prolonged standing or sitting. Movement pain relates to bending, twisting, or lifting, but also to walking, running, reaching overhead, pushing, or pulling, and is claimed as such activities as bed making, vacuuming, ironing, and sexual intercourse.

Did, or does, the pain occur upon arising from a bent-over position? Does lying in a certain position cause pain or relieve the pain? Lying on one's stomach arches the back and may cause sway back pain, which is relieved by changing to a position that decreases the lordosis such as lying on one's side with the knees and hips flexed in the so-called fetal position. Prolonged bent-over posture, however, may cause the pain. Prolonged sitting in a soft chair may cause this type of pain, indicating a flexion cause.

One should be aware that severe injuries are not necessary to cause severe pain to a depressed or frightened person. Pain may be disabling in that it prevents the person from performing activities that are desired, but pain may also be convenient in that undesired activities can be avoided. These reactions may not be intentional or conscious, yet they influence the intensity and severity of the pain.

92

Has the patient been examined, treated, and advised as to the cause and reason for treatment? Too many patients undergo a cursory, unrevealing examination and are given a meaningless *label* of what is wrong. Many receive treatment without knowing why, what is intended, or what is to be expected from that treatment.

Which positions have been advised as desirable and which to avoid? What exercises have been advised, and have they been done properly and conscientiously? What drugs have been tried and with what effect? Have there been side effects from these drugs?

In the final analysis, the patient informs the physician, who in turn should assimilate the stated facts and offer answers to specific questions. Ultimately, the physician should *teach* the patient about the low back problems. **The physician must primarily be a teacher, secondarily a therapist.** Only an informed student can understand cause and effect and the basis of the symptoms and their improvement.

OBSERVATION

The physician learns by observing the patient's posture, movements, and attitude. Posture depicts several possible factors that may be related to the cause of pain.

There are familial traits, such as a round upper back, that can be revealed by seeing other members of the family. A sway back similarly may be noted and be considered normal. The black race notably has a normally accentuated lordosis that is not necessarily painful or disabling.

Mannerisms of the patient are deceptive. They portray the feeling of the patient and convey to the observer what the patient consciously or unconsciously wishes to portray. Severe pain is clearly severe. Movement is clearly limited and is clearly painful. Sitting hurts, standing hurts, or bending hurts. The patient's hand is frequently placed where the pain is.

Body language has become an accepted science in which a person's inner feelings are clearly depicted in posture, movement, or facial expression. This is evident in the patient with low back pain. The assumed posture, the avoided movements, and the grimaces and facial expressions clearly depict the severity, the disabling intensity, and the fear of the consequences of movement or posture.

A visual portrayal of pain and disability may be the only signs of impairment. Everything else in the history and examination may be normal or at least unrevealing. Movement of the patient reveals inability to bend, to turn to the left, to sit, or to lie down. Observing this in the patient aware of being observed, or one unaware of being observed, reveals a great deal about the patient at that moment.

As will be discussed in the chapters on Psychological Factors in Low Back Pain (Chapter 12) and Chronic Pain (Chapter 13), a distinction must be made between what the patient unconsciously reveals, or consciously wishes to portray. The former is a contribution to estimate recovery, whereas the latter may portray inevitable failure of any treatment program.

SPECIFIC EXAMINATION

Posture

The person must be evaluated as to stance, viewed from the side and from behind. Posture must be viewed with the patient aware of being viewed, as this is the posture deemed *by the patient* to be correct or to be causative of pain. The posture that is not consciously assumed is more meaningful.

Does a Posture Cause Pain?

The excessive lordosis noted by the physician may cause more discomfort when accentuated by the examiner. Manually increasing the lordosis may aggravate the pain, whereas decreasing the lordosis may decrease the pain. The opposite effect is also revealing, namely, increasing the lordosis may relieve the pain, whereas decreasing it may aggravate the pain.

Increasing the lordosis and simultaneously bending to the side may increase the pain. By placing the functional unit in this position, it is apparent that the facet joints behind the vertebral bodies come closer together.

In arching backward and bending to the left, the facet joints on the left side come closer together, and the facets on the right side separate. If the facets are damaged, worn, or inflamed as they are brought together and made to bear weight, they may cause back pain. In bending backward and to the left, the left foramen closes and may compress the nerve roots. Pain can result in the back or down the leg on the side of bending. The movement causing pain clarifies the factor that causes the low back pain and/or the leg pain (Fig. 63).

Flexibility

As the patient bends forward, the low back goes from lordosis to the fully flexed-forward position. This requires flexion of each functional unit (8 to 10 degrees). Full flexion means relaxation and flexibility of the

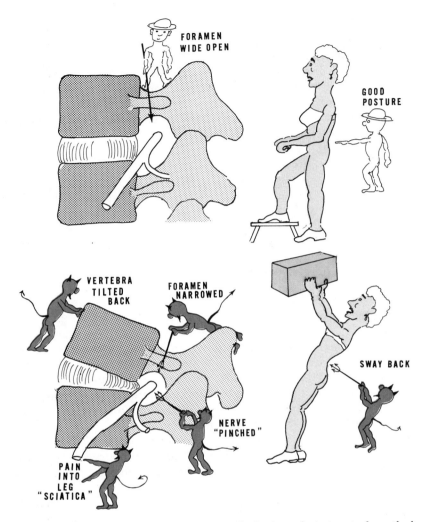

FIGURE 63. Reason a "sway" back can cause low backache *and* sciatic pain down the leg.

muscles and elasticity of the ligaments, fascia, and long ligaments.

How the back bends is more important than *how far* it bends, as is usually denoted by how close to the ground the fingertips reach. Limitation of flexion may result from poor conditioning or from protective guarding by the muscles that refuse to elongate. Failure of the muscle to elongate may mean that the muscles are assuming a protective function in the patient fearing pain by preventing the back from bending.

Flexibility or limitation of low back movement needs to be carefully evaluated. Protective spasm may be unconscious and limit flexion owing

95

to pain from tissue inflammation. Protective spasm may also be incurred by the patient who fears that bending will cause pain or further tissue injury. Differentiating the cause of the spasm may be difficult. A simple way to make this differentiation is to test spine flexion in bending forward from the standing position and in bending forward from the kneeling position. Frequently, spasm from tissue inflammation will be noted from both tests, whereas spasm from fear will be noted in the standing test and not during the kneeling test (Fig. 64).

Re-Extension to the Erect Posture

The person who re-extends normally does so by decreasing the pelvic rotation, then (in the last 45 degrees of re-extension) re-extending and regaining lumbar lordosis (sway). In the painful back, the sway (lordosis) may be regained prematurely, that is, long before the last 45 degrees of full extension or erect posture has been reached. Pain that is experienced during faulty re-extension depicts the mechanism that causes or caused the initial low back pain.

Straight Spine Versus Curved

A person normally should bend down in a straight line. If there is unilateral (one-sided) muscle spasm, the person will stand twisted to that side, or will bend to that side, on attempting to bend forward. The scoliosis, as it is called, may be the result of inflammation of the ligaments or the facets, or of a disk herniation. Functional scoliosis per se does not necessarily indicate a herniated disk. (see Fig. 50).

Lateral bending is rarely limited because of a low back tissue injury. Limitation to either side in addition to forward and backward limitation can depict apprehension and guarding, which cause intentional limitation by the patient.

A person who is scoliotic as a result of one-sided muscle spasm is considered to have functional scoliosis. This scoliosis is noted in the standing erect position and disappears when lying down. A structural curve from gradual bony changes that has its onset in adolescence does not disappear when assuming the vertical position. A structural scoliosis has structural rotation as well as lateral curve. It is visible on x-ray and cannot be corrected by any movement or position.

Tenderness

Pain that is elicited from pressure is termed tenderness. Tenderness usually indicates an injured, stretched, strained, or bruised tissue. The

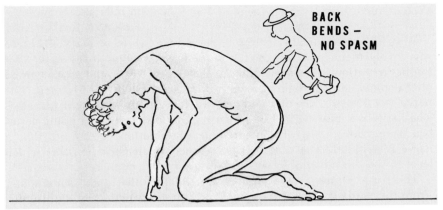

BACK BENDS – NO SPASM

KNEELING TEST

FIGURE 64. Kneeling test. This position helps to differentiate back protection caused by fear from true spasm caused by injury or inflammation.

history reveals the type of injury and the exact site. The point of tenderness indicates the tissue area.

In examining the low back for tender spots, only the muscles and the long ligaments between the bony processes can be palpated. Palpated means available to the touch or pressure of the fingers of the examiner. The facet joints are deep and under heavy muscle. They cannot be directly palpated. Movement of the functional unit by manual pressure from the examiner *assumes* that the pain thus elicited comes from the facets. Tenderness or tender spots felt are usually in the muscles or long ligaments.

Cause of Pain from Inflammation

Pain elicited by a movement or position indicates the position and movement of the functional unit and which tissues are involved. TO CAUSE THE PAIN OR RELIEVE THE PAIN BY SPECIAL MOVEMENT IS THE BOTTOM LINE IN MAKING A PROPER DIAGNOSIS OF WHERE, HOW, AND WHY PAIN OCCURS.

NEUROLOGIC EXAMINATION

Determining whether there is nerve root involvement along with low back pain is important. This constitutes the basis of the neurologic examination.

97

Which Nerve Root? Which Level of The Spine?

Why is it important to determine nerve root involvement? With nerve root involvement, pain may be felt in the legs as well as at the back. This implies irritation of the nerve roots as they emerge from the cauda equina of the spinal cord in their passage to the legs through the foramen. The nerve root passes by the disk and near the facet joints within the foramen. The nerve root may be irritated by a bulging disk or by a slipping vertebra (spondylolisthesis). The neurologic examination determines that a nerve is irritated. The examination reveals which nerve it is, at which level in the lumbosacral spine, and often to what degree it is damaged.

There are relatively few nerve roots related to the lumbosacral spine. From the cauda equina of the spinal cord there are primarily four significant nerve roots.

The third lumbar nerve (termed L_3) passes through the foramen between the third and fourth vertebrae. It then passes down the front of the thigh, carries sensation to the area of skin in front of the thigh, supplies the knee jerk (the reflex elicited by hitting below the kneecap with the rubber hammer), and supplies the muscles of the front of the thigh. This muscle group is used to do deep knee bends and thus is important in climbing stairs, getting out of a chair, and so on. These tests indicate the integrity of L_3.

The fourth lumbar nerve (L_4) passes through the foramen between the fourth and fifth vertebrae. It does not supply a specific group of muscles and does not have a special reflex. It does supply a specific area of skin on the inner side of the lower leg; hence, the doctor diagnoses L_4 damage by testing the skin sensation with a pin, light touch, or a pledget of cotton.

The fifth lumbar nerve (L_5) passes from the lumbosacral spine between the fifth lumbar vertebra and the sacrum. It then passes behind the lower leg into the calf region and carries the sensation of the outer aspect of the calf. It does *not* relate to a specific reflex but does supply one muscle and the major portion of another muscle. The one muscle it controls is the muscle that lifts the big toe, known as the hallucis longus. It also largely supplies the muscle that lifts the foot of the ankle. This latter muscle is called the anterior tibialis and allows a person to walk on the heels or to clear the big toe during walking. A person with weakness of this muscle drags the big toe when walking (see Fig. 58).

The lowest nerve is termed S_1 (first sacral nerve). It leaves the spine through a foramen within the sacrum. It supplies the ankle jerk reflex elicited by the Achilles tendon behind the ankle. This S_1 nerve supplies the sensation of the outer aspect of the front and controls the calf muscle group. Through control of this muscle, a person can rise up on the toes, walk on the toes, jump, and run.

98

There are lower sacral nerves, S_2 and S_3, that control the bladder and convey the sensation around the anus. When these nerves are involved, the person may lose control of the bladder, and occasionally of the bowel, and may lose sensation of the skin of the buttocks.

The neurologic examination thus is important, as the loss of nerve function may cause a loss of function such as walking, stair climbing, running, and so forth. Early or mild pressure on nerve roots may cause pain, tingling, numbness, and fatigue of the muscles. Intense or prolonged pressure on the nerve may cause paralysis or total loss of sensation in the areas of their distribution.

An examination done carefully and precisely reveals the exact level (L_3, L_4, to S_1) and may depict the severity of nerve injury. Further tests become necessary to determine *what* is causing the nerve pressure. *Where* (the nerve root level) has already been established by the neurologic examination described.

CHAPTER 8

Special Tests

WHEN, WHY, AND WHICH?

Many tests of the lumbar spine are of the x-ray variety. These tests reveal what cannot be seen by the eye or felt by the fingers or heard by instruments. X-rays literally reveal what is under the skin and the muscle.

X-rays reveal the size, width, density, and position of the bones. They also reveal the width of the space between bones. In depicting the appearance of the bone, any disease of bones such as metastatic cancer (cancer spread from elsewhere in the body), osteoporosis (decalcification), fracture, or infection changes the appearance of the bones. In demonstrating the space between bones, an x-ray reveals the width of the disk space and the width and integrity of the posterior facet joints.

Surprisingly *little* is learned from the routine x-ray unless a bone disease, congenital abnormality, or injury is suspected. By the age of 50 to 55 years, disk degeneration occurs in most people, causing a narrowed disk space to be noted in most x-rays. This expectedly occurs between the fourth and fifth lumbar vertebrae and between the fifth lumbar and first sacral vertebrae.

People over 50 to 55 years of age often have x-ray evidence of osteophytes, so-called degenerative arthritis with spur formation. Happily, the presence of degenerative changes of the disk need not be symptomatic; if it were, most people in their fifth, sixth, or certainly their seventh decade would have disease with pain and impairment. This condition will be further discussed in Chapter 11.

OSTEOPOROSIS

In postmenopausal women approximately 50 to 55 years of age, bones undergo decalcification. This is called osteoporosis. It does not cause pain but does predispose to softening and therefore to compression fractures, which can be symptomatic.

These conditions, osteophytes or osteoporosis, may be noted in routine x-rays and usually do not change over long periods of time unless there is in addition an acute trauma, injury, intercurrent illness, or an infection. The repeated taking of routine x-rays at each medical visit without a specific indication is to be deplored.

Oblique views, x-ray views of the lumbosacral spine taken at an angle instead of from front to back or from the side, are useful to demonstrate the adequacy of the foramen. These views are important when there is suspicion of narrowing of the foramen, which could encroach upon the nerve roots in their passage through the foramen.

Certain conditions such as spondylolysis (degeneration of joints) are revealed by oblique views. These will be discussed thoroughly in Chapter 11.

The ability of x-rays of the entire spine to demonstrate specific alignment of each vertebra—to show subluxation, off center, minor dislocation, or malalignment—is a misconception. The value of these equivocal changes has been questioned, and the conclusions drawn from these claims border on fancy, not fact.

Too much x-ray exposure has been incriminated as possibly cancer forming, but the exact dosage of x-ray exposure that is dangerous to the patient has not to date been confirmed.

SPECIAL X-RAYS

Myelogram

Myelography is a dye test used to outline any encroachment upon the width and shape of the spinal canal, the foramen, and its contents. Normally, a routine x-ray gives an indication of these abnormalities, but dye injected into the dura specifically outlines the defect. The dura is the sheath of the spinal cord and nerves. It is in essence "the skin of the hot dog." It covers the nerves as a sleeve and contains the spinal fluid that bathes and floats the nerves. Dye is injected into the patient's back with the needle penetrating the dura (Fig. 65).

If there is a disk bulging, an osteophyte protruding, or a tumor of any type within the spinal canal, the dye makes it visible. X-ray after injection of the dye outlines the normal sheath and reveals any encroachment upon it. The type, the size, and the specific level of the defect are visible on myelography to an expert.

There are different dyes. Pantopaque is a heavy oil-base dye that must be removed after the test is over. Metrizamide is soluble and dissolves, thus being excreted or absorbed. If Pantopaque is used, some dye remains in the sac after a myelogram and may remain for years. This has been considered a potential source of chronic irritation. Metrizamide is also

101

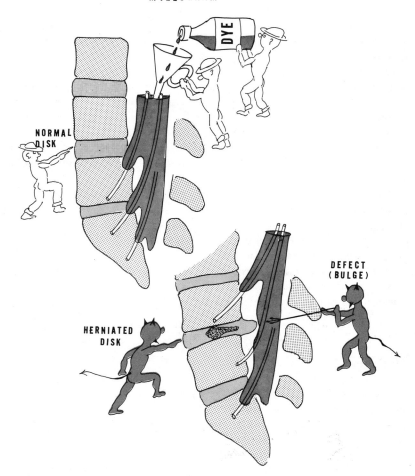

FIGURE 65. Lumbar myelogram: dye test.

irritating but is rapidly absorbed and is brief in its adverse reaction. Metrizamide is a thinner fluid and penetrates further into all of the recesses of the spinal canal than does Pantopaque but requires that the pictures be taken soon after the injection, as the dye may disappear early in the test.

The width of the spinal canal can be determined by myelography. This width is measured between the vertebral body and the lamina. It is the width of the spinal canal through which course the nerve roots. There are standards that determine whether the width is normal.

102

CAT Scan

CAT scan is a computerized axial x-ray in which three views of the spine are simultaneously x-rayed and combined into one picture by a computer. By this highly specialized test all views of the spine may be seen: the front-to-rear view, side view, and top-to-bottom view. Soft, *nonbony* as well as bony aspects of the vertebral column may be visualized.

A bulging disk, a tumor, ligamentous thickening, or bony deformation of the spinal canal may be visualized. This test is new and not yet fully explored, but it may someday replace many of the older techniques. It may replace myelography, but to date both are still frequently used.

NUCLEAR MEDICINE

With the advent of isotopes, a radioactive material is injected intravenously. This material is picked up by tissues that have specific affinity for this material and thus have been tagged by the injected isotope.

If a specific tissue is diseased or is excessive, it will pick up more radioactive dye and be seen on the special camera. Malignancies that have spread to bone, such as from breast, thyroid, or prostate cancer, may be seen in nuclear scans that otherwise would not be seen on plain x-rays or even on CAT scans.

THERMOGRAPHY

Thermography is a recent type of study using a camera that identifies areas of higher or lower temperature on the surface of the body. These images vary on the basis that inflammation requires greater blood supply and higher temperatures are generated in that area. The thermogram reflects this higher temperature by displaying different colors in the sensitive camera film.

These colorful pictures have yet to have an accepted diagnostic value. They do not at this time replace or enhance the other more standardized diagnostic tests.

E.M.G.: ELECTROMYOGRAPHY

E.M.G. is an abbreviation for electromyography. Any nerve that is stimulated by movement voluntarily attempted or electrically stimulated causes a muscle to contract. This contraction can be recorded on a screen similar to a television screen after being transmitted through a needle and wire to the recording machine. A normal nerve to a specific muscle depicts a specific graphic display of a line on the E.M.G. screen. If there is

103

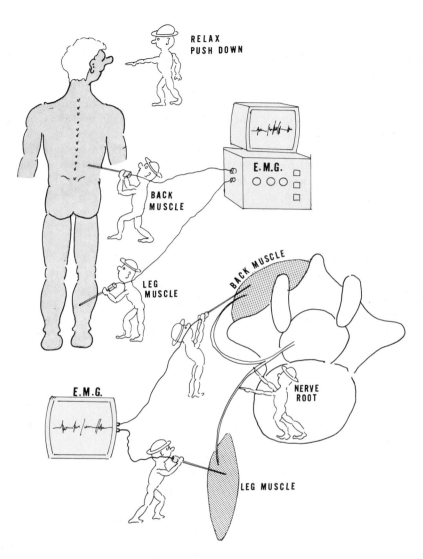

FIGURE 66. Electromyography test to determine "which nerve" and if nerve is damaged or irritated.

abnormality of the nerve, in that it is damaged by pressure, injury, or disease, this will be displayed as being abnormal on the screen (Fig. 66).

An E.M.G. may reveal that conduction of current within a nerve is impaired. By knowing into which muscle the needle is inserted and which nerve furnishes that muscle, the specific nerve that is impaired can be established. As each peripheral nerve contains one or more roots, these specific roots are clearly determined. By testing numerous muscles, the overlapping of their numerous nerves is analyzed until *one* nerve root is implicated. The level of the specific spinal nerve root is established.

It has been shown that a single nerve root emerges from one foramen in the vertebral column; thus, an abnormal E.M.G. identifies the specific foramen.

A nerve under pressure initially does *not* reveal E.M.G. abnormality except for some irritability as the needle enters the muscle. An E.M.G. does not become abnormal until damage has existed for 21 days. An E.M.G. does not specify what is damaging the nerve or the extent of the damage; it merely identifies that there is damage and to which nerve root.

The combination of an E.M.G., a myelogram, and a CAT scan can localize the exact nerve involved and reveal the causative factor.

E.M.G. CONDUCTION TIME

Conduction time may also be tested by a similar E.M.G. type of test. This test shows how rapidly a nerve that has been electrically stimulated conducts that impulse to a specific muscle. That nerve is stimulated electrically and the time is determined from which the stimulus is applied to the instant the muscle contracts. This test is uniquely effective in a diabetic patient or in a person whose system illness causes a decreased nerve conduction.

A damaged nerve or a nerve under pressure may not cause a delay in conduction time if the stimulus is applied distal to the pressure where the nerve conducts the current normally. A conduction time test determines the health of the nerve, not necessarily its integrity. It is of little value in determining root level or the site of spinal pressure.

CHAPTER 9

Treatment

Treatment of the patient who complains of low back pain must have a specific basis for what is recommended. Treatment of the low back with or without leg pain is very similar. The reasons for this will be clarified.

Treatment must be considered for the person who has acute onset of back pain, recurrent episodes of backache, or chronic backache. They are *all* related but have significant differences in regard to treatment.

ACUTE BACKACHE

The dictionary defines *acute* as "severe and sharp: as in pain." In medical terminology, acute means rapid onset of pain and limitation after an activity or situation. From apparent normal painless movement, there is onset of pain with resultant impairment of motion. It may be the first such painful episode.

RECURRENT LOW BACK PAIN

Episodes of pain are reasonably similar in where or how they appear and the manner in which they affect the person. Recurrences may be spaced by years, months, or days. As a rule, a *pattern* may exist in that pain recurs from similar movements or position, or during similar life situations.

CHRONIC LOW BACKACHE

A back pain with or without motion limitation that persists for 3 to 6 months is considered to be chronic. It never leaves completely, although the severity, duration, and region of pain may vary. Often, in chronic pain, the specific movement or position that initially caused or aggravated the pain may become unclear or nonspecific.

The usual recommendations of treatment for a patient with acute low back pain are:

1. Bed rest or at least the reclining position.
2. Medication.
3. Time: How long?
4. Heat or ice to the back.

All these need clarification (Fig. 67).

Effect of Gravity

To eliminate gravity means that once patients have sustained an injury, an acute stress, or an acute episode of irritation to the low back, they must be *off their feet*, not standing or sitting up. By eliminating gravity, pressure is removed from the disk and the joints. Stress on the muscles and ligaments that normally maintain the patient in the erect posture is lessened.

Bed Rest: How?

To eliminate gravity, bed rest is commonly prescribed as the first choice of treatment, with the body placed in the proper position. To say that there is only one position of bed rest, however, is not true because some patients feel comfortable in lying perfectly straight or flat in bed, whereas others feel better in a bent position.

The best tolerated position is usually the bent posture, with the knees slightly bent and the back slightly flexed. The word "slightly" must be stressed; the knees should be bent only slightly, into the position best tolerated by the patient. Proper position of the reclining body allows the irritated tissues to begin recovery.

The bent posture in the usual home bed—hopefully one with a firm mattress—may be accomplished by placing pillows behind the knees (see Fig. 67). It is interesting that placing a large pillow between the knees also tends to maintain the legs in a bent position at the knees and hips. A convenient way of assuring a comfortable bent knee–bent hip position is to place one, two, or three square sofa pillows under the legs. These square pillows stack one upon the other, do not slide, and are a soft acceptable surface under the bent knees. The pillow behind the head may be of any height tolerated by the patient.

107

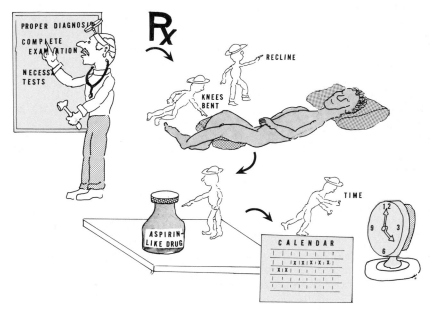

FIGURE 67. Essentials for treating acute low back pain.

Relief of Pain

Pain must be eliminated or reduced early because pain causes the muscles to contract further, that is, go into spasm. The back muscles are already in spasm to prevent movement of the low back. Even though the position of the patient in bed may eliminate or decrease the need for muscle contraction to support the spine, the pain experienced by the patient may cause the muscles to remain in a state of contraction, or spasm.

Pain is usually not severe enough to require strong medicines, but this depends very much on the patient's pain tolerance and the interpretation of the severity of the pain. If the low back pain is localized merely in the region of low back and the cause is known, such as faulty lifting or a twist, home remedies are acceptable. For centuries, patients have been using aspirin or an aspirinlike medicine available over the counter. This is acceptable if this aspirinlike drug is tolerated by the patient. Intolerance is usually manifested by upset stomach, headache, or a rash.

EXTREME SEVERITY, PERSISTENCE OF PAIN IN SPITE OF A BRIEF TRIAL OF HOME REMEDIES, PAIN GOING ELSEWHERE IN THE BODY FROM THE LOW BACK AREA, OR PAIN WITH ANY UNUSUAL SYMPTOMS SHOULD PROMPT CONTACT WITH A PHYSICIAN.

Generally, physicians prescribe pain medication as requested by the patient. Today there are medicines that decrease inflammation and are beneficial in decreasing pain. Most of these drugs are aspirinlike in their action and are known as *nonsteroidal drugs*.

Steroids, or cortisone drugs, are well known to combat and decrease inflammation. By so doing, they decrease pain and limit the duration of impaired mobility. Steroids, however, have potentially severe side effects.

Recently, nonsteroidal drugs have been discovered. These have benefits similar to those of steroids without many of the expected side effects. They do have side effects and should be used by prescription and under supervision of a physician.

An aspirinlike drug does more than decrease the sensation of pain experienced by the patient. It neutralizes the enzymes released in the body by the inflamed tissues. These aspirinlike drugs are neutralizers of the painful tissue substances that cause inflammation. Inflammation in turn may cause pain.

Time for Relief of Low Backache

As inflammation usually requires a certain amount of time before it subsides; 3 to 7 days is the estimated period for most acute problems. This varies, as some patients improve within 1 or 2 days and others have enough inflammation to require even 7 or more days of bed rest.

As has been stated, inflammation is fluid formation in the tissues with toxic substances and possibly microscopic hemorrhaging in the tissues. The skin becomes sensitive. The muscles become irritated and go into spasm. For each of these tissue reactions, there are treatments that have been tested by time and found effective.

Ice or Heat to Back?

Application of ice to the inflamed, tender part is frequently used in tissue injuries anywhere on the body. This also pertains to the low back. To be effective, ice must be carefully applied; it must not merely be placed in a plastic bag and laid upon the back for periods of 20 minutes to 1 hour. Applying ice this way frequently causes more pain and more spasm because ice itself causes the blood vessels of the muscles to constrict. This stops blood flow. Ice used in this way can be irritating.

To be effective, ice is best rubbed back and forth on the skin in slow steady strokes, up and down the skin (Fig. 68). It is best applied by someone other than the patient and should be applied until a pink hue appears in the skin. Ice application for 5 minutes on one side of the back and then on the other side is frequently effective in the early stages of low backache.

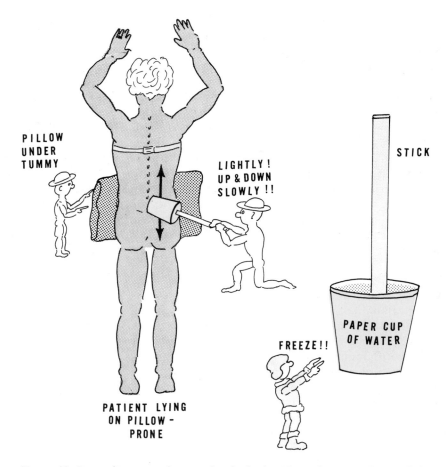

PILLOW UNDER TUMMY

LIGHTLY! UP & DOWN SLOWLY!!

STICK

PAPER CUP OF WATER

FREEZE!!

PATIENT LYING ON PILLOW - PRONE

FIGURE 68. Ice application to the acute low backache. This is done several times daily.

An ice applicator can be easily made. Place water in a paper cup in which a lollipop stick is inserted, then place this in the freezer compartment of the refrigerator to form the applicator. Once frozen, the paper cup is peeled off, and the ice is applied directly to the skin. The person applying the treatment may also hold an ice cube within a small turkish towel washcloth.

When Heat?

Since inflammation is an accumulation of irritating tissue fluids, these tissue irritants must ultimately be dispelled or removed from the inflamed

110

tissues. This is best accomplished by the application of heat, which brings in a new blood supply. This new blood supply eliminates all of the accumulated irritating tissue fluids.

Heat may be applied by hot moist packs or Hydrocollator pads. Hydrocollator pads are chemical pads that are warmed by submergence in hot water and retain the heat for long periods of time. They are usually better tolerated and most effective when wrapped in a towel. Usually a 20- to 30-minute application, two or three times a day, is effective.

The hot pack may be placed *under* the back while the patient is in the flexed position in bed, as previously described (see Fig. 63). If a hot pack is applied to the back with the patient lying on the stomach (the so-called prone position), a large pillow must be placed under the stomach to prevent the back from arching.

ARISING FROM THE LYING POSITION TO THE SITTING AND STANDING POSITION

During the acute phase of low back pain, the patient frequently will have difficulty in getting from the resting, lying position to the sitting or standing position. Resuming the erect position must be done properly during the phase of recovery from the low back acute stress and should be practiced throughout every subsequent day's activities.

The proper way for a person to arise to the sitting then standing position from bed rest must follow this sequence:

1. From the position of lying on the back, the knees are drawn toward the chest.
2. When the knees are at a right angle to the body and the low back is flexed slightly,
3. The person rolls to the side.
4. Now, with the knees and hips flexed and lying on one's side, the person comes to a sitting position *sideways,* using the arms.
5. Once seated with the legs off the edge of the bed, the patient then shifts the center of gravity directly over the knees and feet.
6. The person can now stand up slowly, well balanced over the feet, to the erect position.
7. The erect position need not be fully erect but may comfortably permit only a slightly bent-over position.

Getting back into bed means backing toward the bed. Upon reaching the bed and feeling contact with the bed behind the legs, the following sequence must be followed:

1. Remaining slightly bent forward, slowly sit on the bed.

111

2. Remaining bent over, lie down *sideways* using arm support.
3. Once on the side, still with hips and knees bent, roll over to the back with knees and hips flexed and feet flat to the surface of the bed.
4. At this point, the legs may be slowly straightened to tolerance or replaced back on the pillows.

This manner of leaving and returning to the bed position, as in every other activity, must be properly learned, practiced, and repeatedly used long after the acute episode subsides. This method of arising and reclining prevents recurrence of low backache.

EXERCISE: WHEN AND WHY?

The new blood supply to the inflamed tissues that removes the inflammation comes from the muscles as they contract and relax. Muscles must also contract and relax to massage the fluid out of the inflamed tissues. This eventually relieves pain and ultimately permits greater movement of the back, as the muscles can now elongate. Therefore, along with the application of heat in the early treatment of the acute low back injury, movement of the low back must be instituted as soon as possible.

Movement must be gentle stretching of the tissues that relaxes them. Gently contracting and then relaxing the muscles massages all the tissue fluids out of the area. Pain decreases, function returns, and movement increases.

WHAT KIND OF EXERCISES?

There are two forms of medically approved exercises. These are termed active and passive.

Passive exercise is exercise done *to* the muscles and, therefore, to the patient. Active exercise is done *by* the patient. In *active* exercise, the patient stretches, contracts, and relaxes the muscles. Both types of exercise are necessary, and ultimately, indicated. Passive exercise may also be applied to the patient in the form of massage or stretching.

Massage

Massage is essentially pressure manually applied to the muscles, the skin, and all the tissues between the skin and the muscle.

There are various forms of massage. After pressure is gently, but firmly, applied to the area, the hand moves back and forth in a slow, rhythmic manner in one plane. This plane may be along the spine or away from the spine. The skin moves *with* the hand. This avoids friction, wrinkling, or other stresses to the skin that may produce pain. This movement literally massages the fluid in and out of the inflamed tissue and gently stretches the tissue. By pressure upon the skin, pain is also relieved.

Massage may also be similar to kneading, as one kneads bread. This accomplishes a similar purpose but is not as well tolerated.

Massage may at first be painful since the tissues are irritated but, if gently done, becomes less uncomfortable and is beneficial in decreasing pain and limitation. Massage should be preceded by the application of heat.

Exercises for the Low Back

Exercise is currently considered to be the most important aspect of low back treatment. Exercises have stood the test of time, have proven to be the major beneficial aspect of treatment, and remain the most widely prescribed treatment by the medical profession, the therapist, the gymnast, and others. The type of exercise varies with the physician and with the expected results.

WHAT IS THE PURPOSE OF EXERCISE?

Exercise essentially is aimed at improving the flexibility of the patient, improving the muscle tone, and increasing strength of the patient's back. Exercise also plays a part in improving posture and ensuring the ability of the back to properly bend, stoop, squat, and lift.

HOW DO EXERCISES IMPROVE FLEXIBILITY?

The low back is best stretched by exercise done in the supine, or back-lying, position. In this position, the patient actively stretches his or her own back.

This exercise is done slowly, gently, and repeatedly. The reason for slow, repeated movements is that the soft tissues which must be stretched have an elasticity that responds to gentle, rhythmic stretch and resents forceful violent stretching.

Tissue that is being stretched is like a rubber band. It gradually elongates. A rubber band, however, can tear if it is forcefully, violently, and excessively stretched. Once tissue is torn, it repairs itself with scar tissue that is capable of producing pain. It must be stated clearly and emphatically that properly performed exercise must be done *gently, slowly, repeatedly,* and *persistently.*

With the patient lying in a supine, or back-lying, position, one knee at a time is brought to the chest. A full knee-to-chest position can be accom-

113

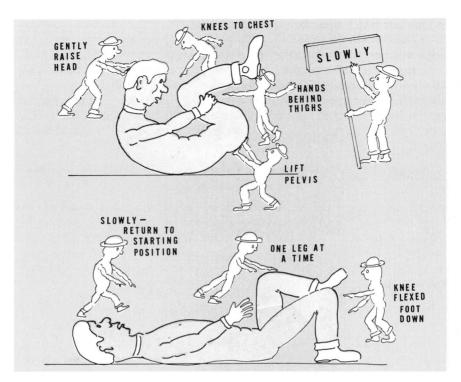

FIGURE 69. Low back stretch (flexibility) exercise. The sequence of this exercise is usually (1) one knee to chest at a time, then (2) both knees. (3) Knees are held to chest for count of five, during which head is raised then lowered. (4) Legs are returned to table *one* at a time.

plished only by the pelvis gradually being elevated from the floor and flexed upon the trunk. In this exercise the leg is used as a lever and must be viewed in this capacity. The patient pulling on the lever must place the hands properly upon the leg (Fig. 69).

If the hand is placed on the front of the lower leg, this forcefully bends the knee upon the thigh. This position of the hand places a great deal of stress upon the knee joint and does not enhance the leverage for stretching the low back. The best position for the hand to pull the knees to the chest is to place them immediately above the knee joint, gripping the back portion of the thigh.

The patient rhythmically brings one knee at a time to the chest and holds it there for a brief period. The *individual* leg is released back to the floor until the foot is flat on the floor. The knee and hip remain flexed. Each leg is flexed individually, then both legs simultaneously. Both knees are brought to the chest wall, held there, then *each leg individually* is released back to the starting position.

114

This last factor must be stressed: namely, releasing the knees from the chest back to the floor *individually*. By lowering one leg at a time, the back will not have a tendency to arch. Bringing both legs down at the same time requires that the hip flexor muscles and the abdominal muscles slowly lower the legs. This is done with some degree of arching of the back. The legs must be, therefore, lowered to the floor individually.

IN SUMMARY: LOW BACK STRETCH

In summary the ideal sequence for exercises to stretch the low back is as follows:

1. Assume back-lying position with knees and hips bent and the feet on the ground.
2. Head is placed in a comfortable position, with or without pillow.
3. Heat is applied to low back.
4. The mind should focus on the exercises, with the intention to be SLOW AND GENTLE.
5. Bring one knee toward chest, placing hands behind thigh slightly above knee joint. Other leg remains as in starting position with foot on ground and hip and knee bent.
6. Slowly, gently, and rhythmically bring knee to chest to *also lift pelvis from floor*. This should give the patient the sensation of the low back being stretched.
7. Once knee reaches chest, it is held for slow count of five.
8. Head is then lifted from floor, held briefly, then lowered.
9. The knee and leg that was bent is returned to the ground as in the beginning. Foot is returned to the ground, but not with leg straight.
10. Other leg is used in the same manner and individually lowered.
11. Both legs are then brought to chest and held, then one leg lowered at a time.

ROTARY STRETCH

The low back must also have some gentle rotatory stretch. This is done in one of two ways.

From the starting position with the feet on the ground and knees and hips bent, the knees are brought (together) toward the chest, then brought to the right (on the left in the other aspect of the exercise), then up to attempt touching the ground at shoulder level, to the side of the body (Fig. 70).) This exercise flexes the low back, then gently rotates (twists) to the right, then the left. The back must remain flexed, thus the

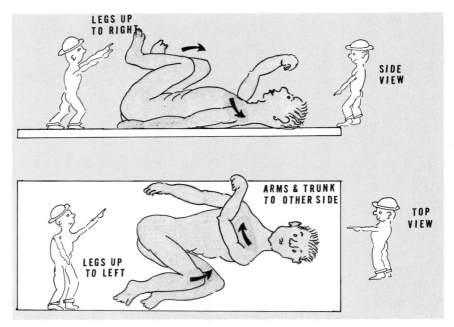

FIGURE 70. Rotatory trunk stretch. With knees flexed toward chest, the legs are slowly lowered to one side, then the other. Arms and upper trunk are rotated to the opposite side. To lower legs when exercise is over, lower one leg at a time.

legs are not first returned to the ground, but merely rotated from right and *up* to left and *up*.

It is the intent of this exercise for the knees not only to be lowered to the side, but at the same time be brought slightly toward the head. The movement of the legs is essentially rotating to the left and slightly upward, then rotating to the right and flexing toward the chest. This must be done slowly and repeatedly. The rotation of the legs rotates the trunk as the shoulders remain on the ground.

When this exercise is finished, with the knees flexed to the chest in the midline, *one leg* at a time is lowered to the floor; as in the previous exercise, each foot is placed on the ground with knees and hips flexed.

This rotating exercise may also be done with the person lying on the back with one foot on the floor and the knee and hip flexed. The opposite leg is brought straight up and pointed toward the ceiling (Fig. 71). In this position, the elevated, straight right leg is lowered to the left side and slightly up toward the shoulder level. Upon returning the leg to the upright position, the knee is bent and the foot is returned to the floor. The opposite leg is then straightened and the same exercise is done on the opposite side.

116

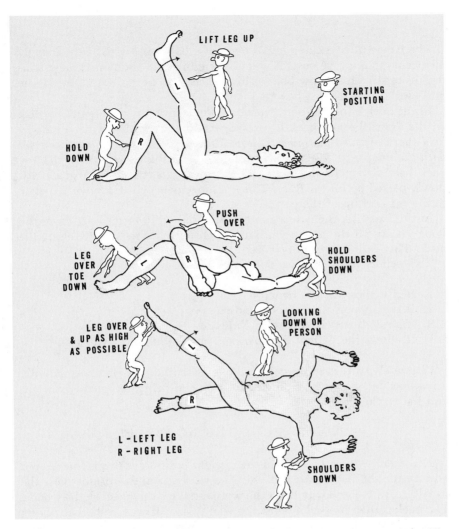

FIGURE 71. Trunk rotatory exercise. The upper picture is the start of the exercise. The middle picture visualizes patient from below, and the bottom picture looks down upon the person. In these pictures, it is the left leg that is raised. Ultimately, both legs are raised.

Throughout these rotatory exercises, the shoulders are kept flat on the floor or the upper trunk can be gently rotated in the *opposite* direction of the rotating legs. Again, the emphasis is on performing these exercises slowly and gently and keeping the back flexed with rest periods between each excursion. In this exercise also, one leg at a time is returned to the starting position.

PELVIC TILTING EXERCISE

The *pelvic tilt*, "tucking in" of the pelvis, is an exercise that is strongly advocated to improve posture and to strengthen the abdominal muscles as well as to stretch the low back. This exercise can be started in the supine position.

In the back-lying position, with both knees and hips flexed and the feet on the floor, the low back is pressed firmly and gently to the floor and *held* there. *At no time must the low back be permitted to leave contact with the floor* (Fig. 72). In the second phase of this exercise with the low back held firmly to the floor, the buttocks (the pelvis) are gradually, slowly picked up off the floor. This is a movement that is known as pelvic tilting, or curl up of the pelvis.

In this exercise, the pelvis can be lifted only a brief distance from the floor, because if the pelvis continues to elevate, it does so by arching the back. This definitely is not desired.

This pelvic tilting exercise does four things:

1. It stretches the low back.
2. It strengthens the buttocks muscles.
3. It strengthens the abdominal muscles.
4. It allows the patient to experience the feeling of pelvic tilting.

Ultimately, this exercise can be done with the legs slowly, gradually extending, but never extending to the point of being completely straight and flat to the floor.

STANDING PELVIC TILTING EXERCISE

This exercise must be done in the upright position as this is the desired posture for the patient to achieve. The patient stands upright with the feet 10 to 12 inches away from the wall and with the knees slightly bent. The back is then pressed against the wall, just as it was in the back-lying exercise in which the back was against the floor. Once the back is pressed against the wall, the pelvis then is slowly peeled away from the wall (Fig. 73), just as it was tilted away from the floor in the back-lying exercise.

THE NEED FOR STRONG ABDOMINAL MUSCLES

It has been stated that "a strong back is a back that has strong abdominal muscles." Why should such a statement be so? The angle of the pelvis determines the lumbosacral angle.

As shown in Figure 23, the *lumbosacral angle* is the angulation of the

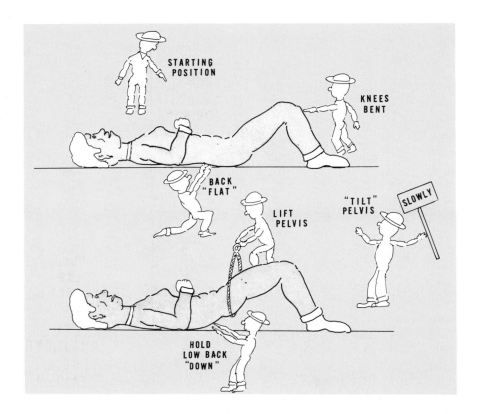

FIGURE 72. Pelvic "tilting" exercise. This is a "flat back" exercise to decrease lumbar lordosis and strengthen the abdominal and buttock muscles. It also teaches this "concept" to the patient.

top surface of the sacrum upon which the lumbar spine is supported. The sacrum is at an angle. The spine supported erect upon the sacrum must be curved to remain above the center of gravity. The greater the sacral angle, the greater the curve of the lumbar spine. The lesser the angle, the lesser the lumbar curve (see Fig. 22).

The pelvis is controlled posteriorly by the buttock muscles that connect to the thigh. The pelvis is also influenced by the upward lift of the abdominal muscles. Posteriorly, the buttock muscles lower the pelvis. Anteriorly, the abdominal muscles elevate the front of the pelvis. Together these muscles determine the angle of the sacrum. This is one of the factors that determine the need for strong abdominal muscles.

It has also been shown that a firm abdominal wall compresses all of the contents of the abdominal cavity. Within the abdominal cavity there is a great deal of entrapped air, both in the bowel and around the bowel, that

119

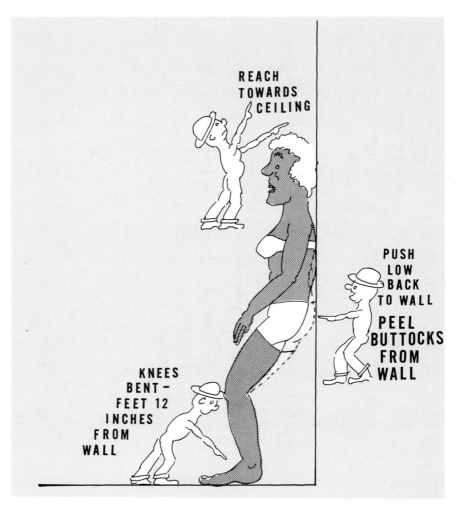

REACH
TOWARDS
CEILING

PUSH
LOW
BACK
TO WALL

PEEL
BUTTOCKS
FROM
WALL

KNEES
BENT –
FEET 12
INCHES
FROM
WALL

FIGURE 73. Pelvic tilting exercise in standing position teaches proper posture and decreases lumbar lordosis.

goes up under the diaphragm and down into the pelvis. This air cavity is contained in the front of the abdominal wall and posteriorly by the lumbar spine, its muscles, and their fascial tissues (the skin of muscles).

As this abdominal cavity is essentially an air-inflated container, it has the tendency to support the spine in the same way an air-inflated bag would support a flexible rod, which in this case is the flexible spine.

It has been shown in medical laboratories that pressure applied against the abdominal wall causes pressure within the abdominal cavity that

120

reduces the pressure of gravity on the spine. The abdominal muscles function in this capacity.

The abdominal muscles also attach to the connective tissues of the ligaments and the fascia of the back and stretch them when the muscles contract. The stretched fascia of the muscles of the back become stronger supporters of the back. Abdominal musculature is thus vitally important in supporting the back.

ABDOMINAL EXERCISES

There are numerous types of abdominal exercises. A word on exercises per se seems indicated. Exercises are either isometric or isotonic. Isometric means the muscle holds but does not shorten or lengthen. In isotonic exercises, the muscle lengthens and shortens. Both increase strength, but isometric exercises presumably increase endurance.

ISOTONIC ABDOMINAL EXERCISES

Beginning with the patient back-lying with knees and hips flexed, the person *slowly* begins sitting up. Curl up is a term used as the person slowly curls up from the floor as if to gradually unpeel the back from the floor. This unpeeling places the intended stress upon the abdominals and avoids any arching.

How far and how frequently the person curls up differs with the individual and his or her physical conditioning. At first, curling up a few degrees, then holding (isotonic to isometric), and then slowly returning to the lying position may be all that can be tolerated or even possible.

Sets, the term athletes use to specify the number of exercises done, vary but should start with a few and gradually increase. *Speed is neither recommended nor beneficial.* Rest between sets is valuable.

Ultimately, a person may come to a complete sit up, from lying to nose reaching the knee.

ISOMETRIC ABDOMINAL EXERCISE

A variation of this ISOTONIC ABDOMINAL EXERCISE is to add isometric exercise. Isometric exercise adds endurance to muscles as isotonic exercise adds strength. To add the isometric exercise, the person sits up, that is, curls up a few degrees and *holds there*, then slowly returns down. The duration of holding may at first be brief, but as the person gains strength and endurance the time increases.

REVERSE ISOMETRIC ABDOMINAL EXERCISES

Early in reconditioning a poorly conditioned individual, the reverse of the isometric abdominal exercise just described is advisable (Fig. 74). In this exercise the person begins with hips and knees bent and the back flexed in the fully bent-forward posture, that is, nose to knees. The person now slowly leans back from this flexed position, approximately 30 to 40 degrees and **holds**. After a period of holding, the person returns to full sitting position.

WHERE ARE THE ARMS HELD?

All the abdominal exercises described can be done with the arms in different positions depending upon the condition of the person. With arms in front of the body or with the hands behind the head and elbows in front, there is less demand upon the abdominal muscles. As the elbows go back behind the head with the hands behind the head, there is more demand placed upon the abdominal muscles.

The purpose of abdominal exercise is to strengthen and increase endurance *at the pace* and *tolerance* of the individual.

There does not seem to be any rationale for going all the way back from the upright flexed position to the full back-lying position and sitting up again to strengthen the abdominal muscles. Although this is not contraindicated, only after the patient has regained sufficient strength can this exercise be done without back strain and does it become permissible.

OBLIQUE ABDOMINAL MUSCLE EXERCISES

There are muscles in the abdomen that not only flex but also rotate the trunk. These are the oblique muscles. They must be strengthened. The exercise to do this consists of leaning back no farther than the 25 or 30 degrees as in the isometric exercises, then slowly turning the body to the right and holding.

After a brief period of holding in this position of leaning back with trunk turned to the right, the person returns to facing forward but *still* leaning back. Then the person, still leaning back 25 to 30 degrees, turns to the left and holds. Finally, the person returns to midline and fully sits up (Fig. 75). Rest and repeat.

SUMMARIZATION OF EXERCISES

Exercises should be initially to stretch, that is, to increase flexibility, but simultaneous exercises should also increase strength and endurance. The

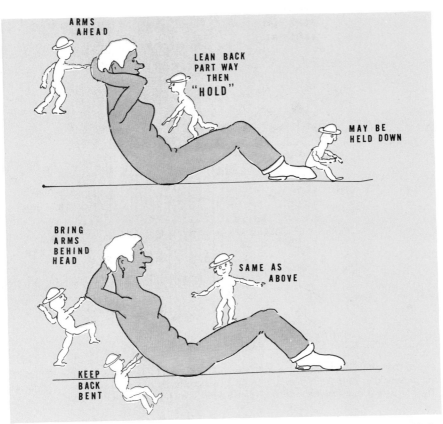

FIGURE 74. "Reverse isometric" abdominal exercises. Person "leans" back about 25 to 30 degrees, then "holds." This contracts abdominal muscles. At first, arms with hands behind head are held in front of body. Gradually, arms are brought "behind" the head. This increases the demand on the abdominal muscles. Hold briefly at first, then longer, to tolerance.

easiest ones should be done first and the more difficult ones gradually undertaken.

HASTE MAKES WASTE. Progressing too fast may bruise or injure muscles, delaying total recovery.

WHAT ABDOMINAL EXERCISES NOT TO DO

Straight Leg Raising

A standard form of exercise to strengthen the abdominal wall has been to lie on the back, then raise both legs off the floor (Fig. 76). *This is not a*

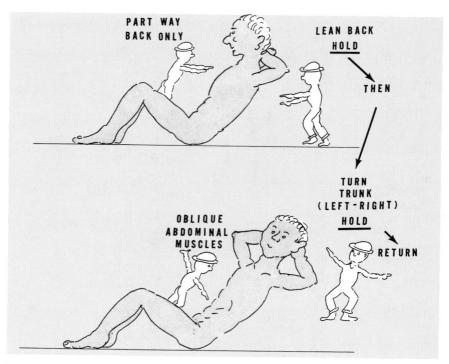

FIGURE 75. Oblique abdominal muscle exercise. This exercise begins as noted in Figure 74, but once held at 25 to 30 degrees, the trunk is rotated, held, then returned to straight ahead. The one arm comes forward and the other behind. Trunk must remain "flexed."

good exercise. It especially must not be done if backache is felt while doing the exercise or after having done this exercise.

As one lifts both legs simultaneously, unless the abdominal wall muscles are extremely powerful, this exercise cannot be done without arching the back. The back arches because the legs are lifted by muscles known as the hip flexors. These hip flexors attach to the front part of the thighs and also to the front of the lumbar spine. Lifting both legs at the same time increases the lordosis of the low back. Consequently, a straight leg raising exercise in which both legs are raised at the same time with the knees fully straight is *not* good for the low back or the abdominal muscles.

Sit-Ups with Legs Straight

Exercise with the trunk coming up from the back-lying position to the sit-up position with the knees straight is also *not* good. With the legs held straight, most of the trunk begins its lift from the floor by the hip flexors (Fig. 77). There is a slight instance of arching the back during the sit-up

124

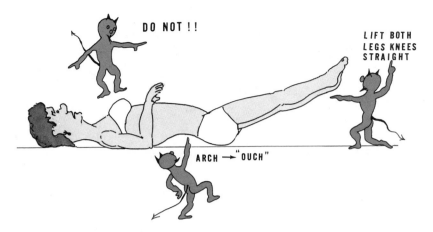

FIGURE 76. Straight leg raising is *not* advised. Straight leg raising tends to arch low back, which is a no-no.

that can produce pain. Until the abdominal musculature becomes strong enough to permit this exercise, it should be done with the knees and hips flexed and the feet flat on the ground as shown in Figure 70.

A sit up from the full back-lying position to a full sit-up position may be done when the abdominal muscles are sufficiently strong (Fig. 78). It must, however, always be done with a gradual curling of the back, which prevents the back from arching.

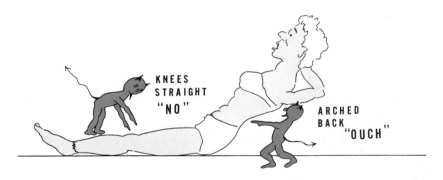

FIGURE 77. Wrong abdominal exercise. Situps with legs straight are a no-no. In this exercise, there is a tendency to arch the low back.

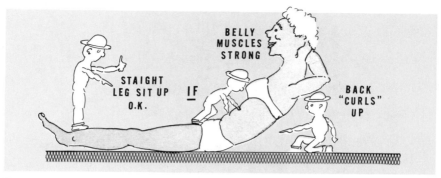

FIGURE 78. Situp with legs straight. This is permitted *only* if abdominal muscles are strong enough to permit patient to *curl* up and back and *not* arch low back.

EXTENSION EXERCISES

Should back exercises only be to flex (bend) the spine, or should they be to extend (arch) the spine? Which is normal?

A flurry was created in the recent decade by a claim made that the extended (arched) spine is normal and that most, if not all, people would lose their backaches by regaining and maintaining the arched (sway) back. Is the arched back normal? Do people get backache by flexing the spine? Do people with low backache benefit from maintaining an arched back? Yes and no! Some people benefit and others suffer from arching the low back (Fig. 79). Some benefit from decreasing the lordosis.

Who Should Arch the Low Back?

Which is proper? Who should flex? Who should arch? Are *all* people the same?

Patients whose low backs are subjected to prolonged excessive forward flexion, either in their daily professions or due to their daily postural habits, possibly *overstretch* the tissues of the lumbar spine, and hence overstretch the posterior tissues of their functional units.

Visualize the excessively and persistently flexed spine and thus flexed functional units. The posterior superior ligament, the muscle sheath, the posterior long ligament, and conceivably the posterior annular fibers—all sensitive—can be excessively stretched (see Figs. 32 and 33).

Pain can result. This type of injured patient is one who works slumped forward, sits slumped forward, or has sustained an acute or repeated flexion injury. This patient develops low backache from being in the flexed position.

126

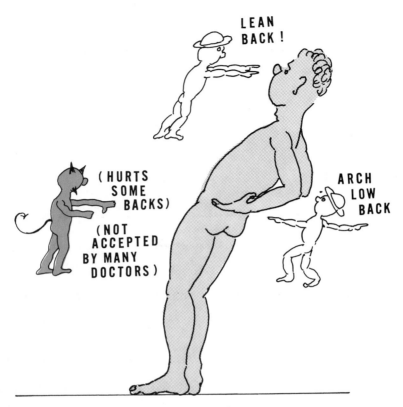

LEAN BACK!

(HURTS SOME BACKS)

(NOT ACCEPTED BY MANY DOCTORS)

ARCH LOW BACK

FIGURE 79. Painful low back arch. Some patients lose backache when arched. Most get low backache with excessive arch. Person's response must be determined in order to advise extension exercises or not.

Examination of this patient reveals excessive and painful forward bending of the low back. These people also often have tight hamstrings. These are the muscles behind the thighs that prevent forward bending or restrict straight leg raising. As a rule, x-rays are not helpful in diagnosis.

Pain in this condition is felt in the mid-low back area, and the tissues there are often tender to pressure. Pain is relieved by arching the back.

TREATMENT USING EXTENSION OF LOW BACK

Treatment is to prevent further stretching of the already overstretched tissues. This is done by arching the low back and keeping it in that position throughout the waking hours. This can be done by exercises, by posture training, or by supporting the back in an arched position.

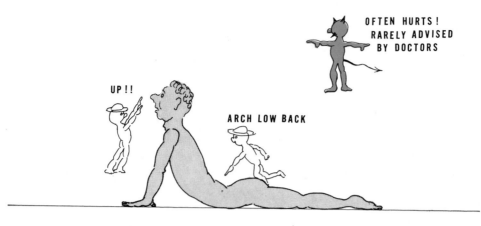

OFTEN HURTS!
RARELY ADVISED
BY DOCTORS

UP!!

ARCH LOW BACK

FIGURE 80. Position to "relax" low back that has been held too long in a bent-over position.

Patients with low back pain relieved by regaining their sway backs may be given the following advice:

1. Sleep on the stomach.
2. Spend long periods of time lying on the stomach supported on the elbows.
3. From this position, patients increase their lordosis by remaining on the stomach and straightening the arms. They are thus prone but up on their hands with elbows extended (Fig. 80).
4. They are advised to sit with a rolled pillow at the base of the low back to arch the low back.
5. Frequently during the day they should stand with the back arched.
6. Avoid any exercise or activity that flexes the low back.

It is obvious that only a certain percentage of patients fit this category. When a patient does fit, the treatment is obvious: arch the low back (Fig. 81).

A person who maintains the arched position too long may ultimately adjust to this position. The low back tissues that had been considered overstretched and the cause of pain now become shortened and become painful when stretched even when they are very slightly stretched. This type of low back pain patient now does *not* reverse lordosis on attempting forward bending. The low back does not bend, and when bending is attempted, the patient gets pain. Gentle low back stretching must now be added to the daily exercise program, but the daily posture must remain arched.

128

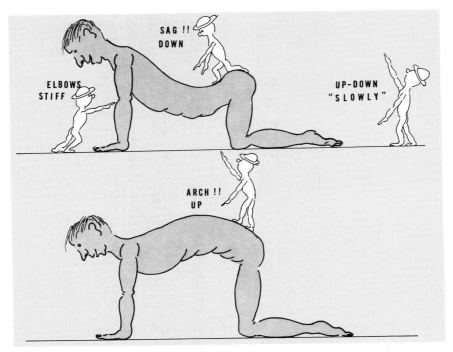

FIGURE 81. In the upper picture, the patient "arches" the low back. In the lower picture, he flexes the back, strengthening abdominal and buttock muscles.

Although there is a fine line of differentiation, the position or the movement that causes pain must be determined. If lordotic posture affords relief, it must be learned. If this posture prevents free bending forward, it must be corrected.

No two patients are alike. No two patients, therefore, routinely receive the same advice.

LATERAL FLEXION EXERCISES

As shown in the first chapter, the back muscles attach to the transverse processes of the functional unit. These attachments are to the *sides* of the spine; thus when the muscles shorten, they bend the spine to the side as well as arch it backward (Fig. 82). By this side attachment, they must also relax and stretch to permit side bending (Fig. 83).

Exercises must be performed to permit this movement. When the legs are spread slightly and the person is erect, one arm can reach down the side of the leg while the other reaches over the head to the same side (Fig. 84).

129

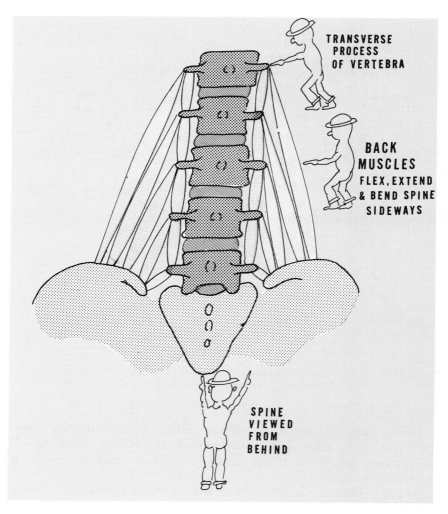

TRANSVERSE
PROCESS
OF VERTEBRA

BACK
MUSCLES
FLEX, EXTEND
& BEND SPINE
SIDEWAYS

SPINE
VIEWED
FROM
BEHIND

FIGURE 82. Extensor muscles that all bend the spine laterally (to the side).

When this exercise is done slowly with gradual increase in stretch, the lateral back muscles and their coating (fascia) elongate. This improves the flexibility in side bending.

The lateral muscles also must be strong. This strength can be gained by flexing laterally against some resistance. One exercise to do this is to stand balanced on one leg, then slowly raise the opposite leg to the side as far as it will go, hold, then slowly lower to the floor (Fig. 85). A weight attached to the ankle increases the resistance.

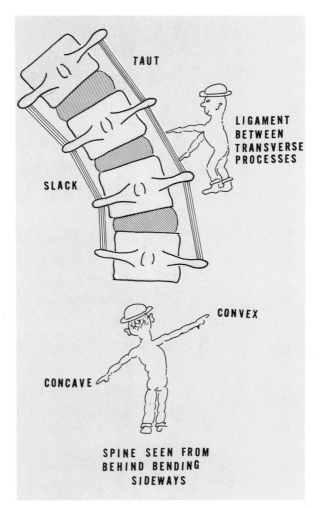

TAUT

LIGAMENT
BETWEEN
TRANSVERSE
PROCESSES

SLACK

CONVEX

CONCAVE

SPINE SEEN FROM
BEHIND BENDING
SIDEWAYS

FIGURE 83. Lateral ligaments of the spine. These lateral ligaments allow side bending but must be kept flexible by exercise (see Fig. 84).

TRACTION: WHEN, HOW, AND WHY?

Numerous other forms of treatment will stretch the low back muscles to the degree that muscles can be stretched by exercise. These forms of stretching are essentially traction. Traction is passive stretching of the low back muscles and ligaments done by the patient or to the patient.

There are numerous methods by which traction is applied to the back. The simplest form is lying on the back with the hips and knees flexed and

131

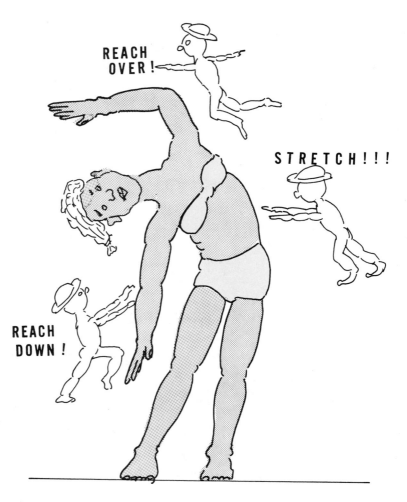

REACH OVER!

STRETCH!!!

REACH DOWN!

FIGURE 84. Side bending exercises. This exercise *gently* stretches the spinal muscles (see Fig. 82) and ligaments (see Fig. 83). Exercise must be done *slowly* and *gently*.

with the legs up on a chair, well supported by a pillow suspending the body off the floor (Fig. 86). This is based on the same principle of traction that is applied to a patient admitted to a hospital for traction.

Traction can be applied with a canvas cloth sling that is attached to the pelvis by a series of straps and weights (Fig. 87). This is the usual method employed in a hospital but can also be used in the home.

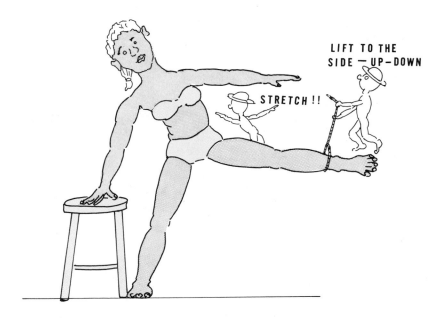

LIFT TO THE
SIDE — UP–DOWN

STRETCH !!

FIGURE 85. Side bending exercise. This exercise strengthens the side-back muscles (see Fig. 82) and the lateral thigh muscle. The leg must *not* be brought *backward* too far, as that would arch the low back.

Gravity Traction

More recently, a recommendation has been made that the person use his own body weight and dangle from either the arms or the feet and allow gravity to be the source of traction to the spine.

Traction here is based on the principle that the body weight uses gravity to stretch the spine. In this type of traction (Fig. 88), the body may merely hang or the patient may perform exercises while in traction.

Exercises done within these various forms of traction are considered beneficial. The muscles contract, relax, decrease the lordosis, and stretch the muscles. The muscle sheath, known as fascia, and the ligaments get stretched while gravity is eliminated.

If traction has been beneficial it may be so for only brief periods. The patient ultimately must resume the erect posture: standing, sitting, walking, bending, and stooping. Thus, traction must be supplemented with every other aspect of low back care, such as exercise.

133

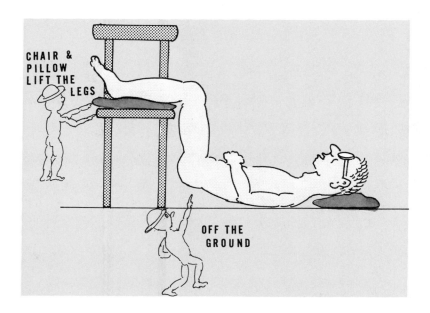

FIGURE 86. Pelvic traction. By placing legs on chair and sufficient pillows, the body is lifted from the floor. This flexes and stretches the low back. Remain in this position as long as possible.

IS A CORSET INDICATED? WHEN? WHAT TYPE?

Occasionally, a person who has a minor defect in the back and/or who has had recurrences of back insult may benefit from the use of a corset, or a back support.

There are many concepts about corseting, but the principles are the same. A back support must essentially achieve the following objectives:

1. The back must be restricted from excessive bending, extending, or twisting.
2. The proper posture must be maintained in that the sway must be decreased with the pelvis tucked in or tilted.
3. The abdomen must be tucked in so that the low back is flat (Fig. 89).

These three objectives outline the purpose of the corset: proper posture, muscle tone, and proper conditioning.

A corset, therefore, has value in that it ensures that the patient bends, sits, or stoops with the back held in the proper position. It prevents exces-

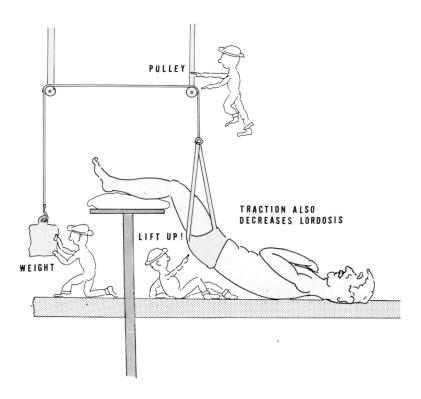

PULLEY

TRACTION ALSO
DECREASES LORDOSIS

LIFT UP!

WEIGHT

FIGURE 87. Hospital-type pelvic traction. Weight varies from 20 to 60 lb as tolerated by patient and indicated by patient's size and weight.

sive bending. The corset also substitutes for the abdominal muscles in keeping the abdomen flat and the low back flat.

Ultimately, a corset can defeat the purpose for which it was given by allowing all of the tissues that normally would do this to become lazy. Muscles that are not used lose their strength and their endurance. Ligaments that are not stretched gently and placed under some degree of tension lose their elasticity and their support. Also, the mind that is not trained to maintain proper posture and maintain proper function becomes lazy from relying on the corset.

The corset can be a friend at the beginning and an enemy in the future. A corset must always be considered a means to an end. In addition to being properly corseted, the patient must be simultaneously placed on a program of exercise and trained in correct posture and activities.

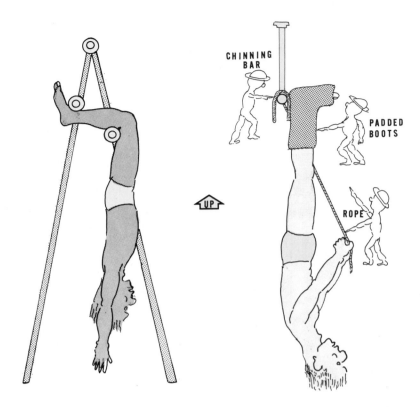

FIGURE 88. "Gravity" traction. There are numerous types of equipment for this traction—hanging from feet via boots or from the knees. The principle is that the weight of the upper body stretches *all* the tissues of the low back: the muscles, fascia, ligaments, and possibly the disks.

WHAT DOES MANIPULATION DO?

Manipulation has been used for centuries in an attempt to relieve low back pain. It is reported to be successful in a certain number of patients. No one fully understands what manipulation does, or where, why, or when it works. There are many explanations offered, a few of which will be discussed.

Manipulation implies a force imposed upon the musculoskeletal system to cause rotation and traction. In this text, manipulation applies to treatment of the low back.

The force needed for manipulation can be what is called long lever or short lever. In the long lever, the leg acts as the lever and the patient lying

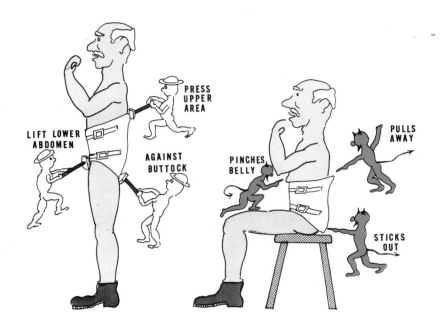

FIGURE 89. Lumbosacral corset. Figure at left shows desirable features of corset, but there are also undesirable (figure at right) features of most corsets.

on the side has the pelvis rotated upon the spine via the leg. In a short lever, the hands of the manipulator are applied directly to the pelvis or the spine. After the spine is fully rotated, a brief thrust, considered to be of high velocity through a brief distance, is applied. The thrust rotates *and* elongates the spine on that side (Fig. 90).

When manipulation is accepted by a patient, *it must be gentle* and precise and must not be done when there is the possibility of damage or pressure upon the nerve roots. Manipulation must not be done when bones or joints are diseased and could be further damaged by manipulation.

One of the theories of benefit from manipulation is that it unlocks joints of the spine. Only the facet joint can conceivably be locked, but this has yet to be proven. The intervertebral disk cannot be returned to its central position between the vertebrae, so the disk is not the tissue that is manipulated.

The tissue that is probably most affected by manipulation is the muscle of the functional unit. If the particular functional unit of the spine has become irritated or inflamed by an improper movement or position, it

137

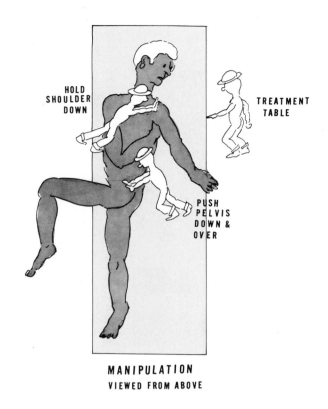

HOLD
SHOULDER
DOWN

TREATMENT
TABLE

PUSH
PELVIS
DOWN &
OVER

MANIPULATION
VIEWED FROM ABOVE

FIGURE 90. Rotatory manipulation. This technique is considered "global" in that the entire body is rotated, the pelvis in one direction and the shoulders in the other direction. The effect is *not* on a specific vertebra or functional unit.

may become splinted by muscle spasm. During manipulation, the muscle is placed on stretch as far as it can be, then given a further stretch as a thrust. This thrust movement is usually one of rotation applied to the flexed spine. This particular position stretches the back muscles. When the muscles are stretched, both the long fibers and the spindle fibers are stretched (see Fig. 24). The thrust then actually further acutely stretches the spindle, which releases the spasm. Movement of the functional unit returns.

That the muscle spindle spasm is released by manipulation is purely hypothetical but appears feasible, as it is based upon the same principle as is stretch by exercise or by traction. This principle could explain why manipulation, preceded by hot moist packs, massage, or stretch, so suddenly decreases the back spasm and relieves pain. Deep muscle massage

138

and stretching by various techniques frequently achieves the same beneficial result.

Another basis for implicating the muscle as the tissue affected by manipulation is that frequently after successful manipulation, or adjustment, there is a return of spasm with low back pain when the patients resume sitting, standing, walking, or bending.

Another plausible explanation for the reason manipulation decreases spasm and unlocks the joints of the spine may be its effect upon the capsule of the joint.

Every joint of the body considered to be a synovial joint must have:

1. A capsule surrounding the joint that contains
2. Joint lubricating fluid and
3. Cartilage coating each opposing bone surface that forms the joint.

The capsule is thin, reasonably elastic, and waterproof, that is, it does not leak out the fluid. The facet joints of the spine are synovial joints.

Joint capsules are supplied with different types of nerves. Type I and Type II nerves act reflexly by going to the spine from the capsule, then connecting to other nerves in the cord to return to the muscles in the same vicinity of that specific joint. They theoretically can either relax or contract these muscles. Type III nerves from the capsule carry the sensation of pain.

Injury to the spine thus injury to the facet joint may have irritated the capsule and thus irritated the Type I and II nerves, resulting in spasm. Manipulation may interrupt this cycle by stretching the capsule. This in turn causes the muscles to relax.

This explanation may account for the quick relief of spasm and the almost immediate return to movement of the spine after a manipulation. Manipulation may have abruptly stretched the capsule. This theory also explains why, shortly after manipulation, spasm and scoliosis may return. The capsule tissues of the facets have remained irritated and thus have remained susceptible to a return of the protective spasm.

This theory also explains why exercise, proper alignment, and proper training in normal spine function are necessary to overcome the acute painful condition and prevent recurrences.

Repeated manipulations are to be condemned if they are not accompanied by the entire treatment program. Manipulation, to be successful, should be accompanied by exercises, improvement of posture, and correction of other mechanical factors. Manipulation must be considered to be another form of treatment used to release muscle spasm that has occurred to splint the inflamed tissues of the functional unit.

If the value of manipulation is based on muscle stretching, it stands to reason that the functional unit of the lumbar spine can now flex and return to full erect posture. As stated in Chapter 1, it must be remembered that the spine flexes forward as the back muscles elongate and returns to the erect stance as they shorten. Without the flexibility the spine cannot function.

It cannot be stressed too much that the manipulation must always be done carefully, gently, and precisely. Manipulation must always also be followed by other methods considered to be necessary to realign the body in posture, regain flexibility, and be normal in everyday functions.

WALKING: GOOD OR BAD?

Brisk walking, while swinging the arms and swaying rhythmically from side to side, stretches and strengthens the lateral trunk muscles. It is good and to be recommended (Fig. 91).

IS RUNNING OR JOGGING GOOD FOR THE BACK?

For the person who has no low backache or is not prone to have repeated low backaches, running or jogging for other health reasons is acceptable.

The person who has recurrent or persistent low backache should *not* run or jog. Slow running (jogging) is done with a degree of lordosis and with the body slightly ahead of the center of gravity. Each step of the leading leg in jogging jars the back with an impact of many times the body weight. Running faster than a jog decreases the frequency and duration of the leading leg striking the ground hard. In running, the foot usually lands on the toes and not the heel, thus minimizing the jar. Running is acceptable unless, as the person fatigues, the running converts to jogging.

It can be said that running is permitted but is not an exercise prescribed for the patient with low back pain.

RECURRENT LOW BACKACHE

Once the patient with the acute onset of low back pain has recovered and strength and flexibility have been regained by the proper exercises, every attempt must be made to prevent recurrence. The flexibility of the back, both in flexion and lateral (side) bending, must be regained and maintained. *Exercises must become a way of life.* Strength of the muscles also must be maintained.

Now we must guard against using the back improperly to prevent another injury. Proper posture, which has been discussed in Chapter 3, must be gained and retained. Proper sitting and standing must be practiced until they become automatic. This also was discussed in Chapter 3.

140

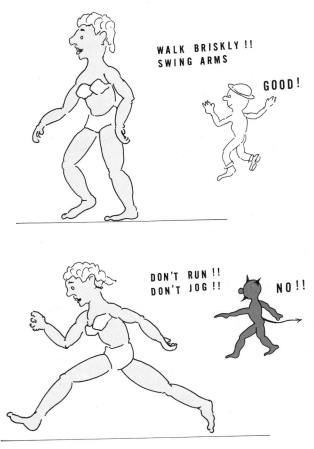

FIGURE 91. Walking: good. Jogging: bad. Running: acceptable.

THE WRONG WAY TO BEND AND LIFT

Improper bending and lifting, as was noted in Chapter 3 as a cause of low backache, must be avoided. Since this function, done improperly, is such a frequent cause of low backache and low back injury, further discussion seems indicated. Please, however, review Chapter 3, then read on.

MAKING USE OF THE STRENGTHENED MUSCLES

All of the strengthening of the abdominal muscles, be they the flexors (benders) or the obliques (rotators), and the stretching of the low back are of no significant value if the back is not properly used.

141

Body Mechanics: The Back School

Teaching and training the individual in the proper use of the back are known as body mechanics. This is the intent of the currently advocated programs of *The Back School*. The Low Back School teaches the patient how to use the back properly.

The school teaches proper posture. It teaches the person how to bend, stoop, squat, and resume the erect position properly. It teaches the person how to bend and lift properly. It also teaches the person what *not* to do that can cause back pain, strain, and stress with injury.

Bending Properly

As stated in the first chapter, a person stands fully erect with muscles of the back relaxed and the ligaments of the back relaxed. The back is supported by the pressure within the disks. Proper erect posture requires essentially no effort. As the person starts to bend forward, as in reaching down to pick something from in front of the body, or to touch something in front of the body, the back muscles immediately contract the very instant the person leans slightly forward, ahead of the center of gravity.

As shown in the first chapter, these very small and very powerful muscles are attached from transverse process to transverse process, allowing the posterior superior spines to open. Each functional unit bends approximately 8 degrees, then the muscles stop elongating. This slow elongation of the erector muscles keeps the functional unit from flexing rapidly.

These muscles gradually elongate and slowly decelerate the amount and speed of bending of the spine. The speed of muscular elongation determines the rate at which the spine bends. Slow flexion of each functional unit to 8 degrees of flexion allows the lumbar spine (five functional units) to bend approximately 45 degrees from the erect lordotic posture. This means that as a person bends forward the lumbar spine (low back) bends to 45 degrees without needing any movement of the pelvis about the hip joints. Each of the five units forming the lumbar spine must bend about 8 to 10 degrees. To permit this flexion, the muscles must be flexible and must be trained to elongate slowly and smoothly. This is a matter of exercise and training.

After the lumbar spine becomes flexed to 45 degrees, the pelvis—upon which the spine is balanced—gradually and slowly must rotate. This pelvic rotation occurs about the hip joints. Both the pelvis rotating about the hip joints and the low back bending forward occur simultaneously until the person has fully bent forward.

At this point of total flexion, the lumbar spine and the pelvis, all of the tissues of the pelvis, the back of the thigh muscles, and the low back have now stretched as much as they can. Bending forward stops at this point.

142

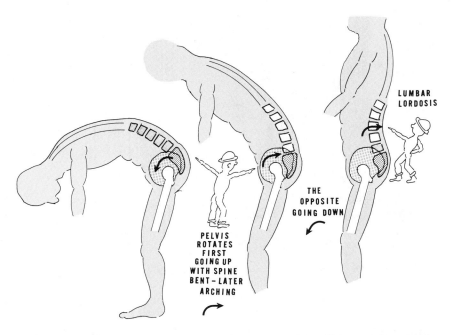

FIGURE 92. Stages of proper re-extension from bent-over posture to 45 degrees of re-extension. The lumbar spine remains flexed. Only the pelvis derotates. At 45 degrees, the lumbar spine regains its lordosis.

RE-EXTENSION TO THE ERECT POSITION

The person who has bent over must come back to the fully erect position. This must be done in a symmetric, synchronous way, performed exactly the opposite way the back and pelvis moved in bending forward. Returning to the erect position is done with the back remaining bent forward while the pelvis rotates about the hip joints. The pelvis continues to rotate until the lumbar spine is still bent about 45 degrees ahead of the center of gravity. At this point of re-extension, and only at this point, does the lumbar spine now start recurling into the lordotic position.

To regain the lumbar lordosis, the muscles of the back, which have up to now been used passively, must shorten to bring the transverse processes and the posterior spines together. Regaining lordosis is done in the last 45 degrees of re-extension. Once the spine has become fully erect, the pelvis has totally derotated and the lumbar spine has regained its lordosis (Fig. 92).

Low Back School trains the patients to do this re-extension properly. Re-extension to full erect posture is performed with the knees bent. This

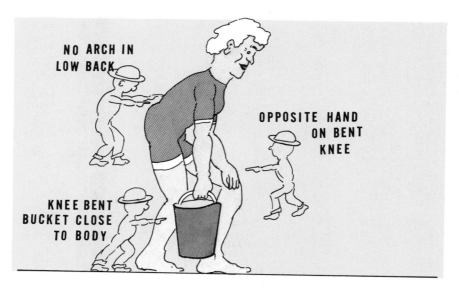

FIGURE 93. Proper one-arm lift.

permits the pelvis to rotate and derotate more efficiently than if the legs were straight.

Also in picking up an object, or assuming that an object is being picked up, when the spine returns to the erect position, whatever is being picked up must be picked up close to the body. It must also be picked up directly in front of the body (Fig. 93).

SHOULD THE SPINE TWIST IN BENDING AND RE-EXTENDING?

Bending should always be in a straight forward-and-back direction without any degree of turning, twisting, or rotation. The reason for bending forward in this manner is that the alignment of the facet joints permits essentially only the movements of bending and re-extending and allows no turning or twisting.

Once we are bent forward we can, however, slightly twist to the right or to the left and rotate the spine (Fig. 94). This places the spine in an asymmetric alignment. As the spine retains the erect position from being bent forward with some rotation, if it does not *derotate* symmetrically and synchronously, the joints in the back are thrown out of line. This improper circuitous return to the erect posture can cause the facets to become impinged.

144

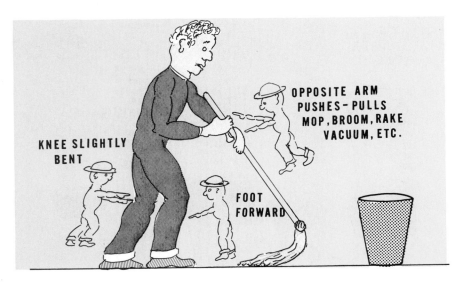

FIGURE 94. "Diagonal principle" of proper mopping, vacuuming, raking, and so forth.

MOST COMMON CAUSE OF LOW BACK INJURY

Bending forward and attempting to regain the erect position improperly when the body has turned and twisted to the right or to the left of the midline is one of the most common causes of back injury.

In addition to improper derotation, if the spine regains its lordosis before it has reached the 45 degrees of flexion upon re-extension, further injury can result. Consequently, the Low Back School teaches the person to pick up objects from the floor or a table ahead by merely bending forward and re-extending in a straight line without rotation and not by regaining the lordosis of the back before re-extension to the 45 degrees of bent forward posture has been reached (Fig. 95).

PROPER LIFTING

Lifting an object properly requires that the mind and the body be oriented as to the size and weight of the object, the distance that the object must be lifted, and where and to what position and direction the object must be placed. If the mind is properly oriented, although it is a momentary decision, it is doubtful that the body would misdirect this task.

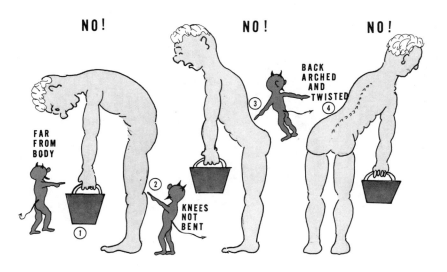

FIGURE 95. Improper aspects of lifting that can injure the low back: (1) Object lifted far from body; (2) lifting without bending knees; (3) regaining lordosis prematurely; (4) bending and twisting and returning to erect position improperly.

Once the size, weight, direction, and speed of lifting the object are determined, the object must be lifted directly in front of and close to the body. Once the body has fully straightened as much as is needed with the object lifted close to it, the entire body can then turn to place the object where it will eventually be deposited.

If the object that is being lifted is heavy, the person should walk around in that direction rather than twist the body. If the object is acceptably light, the body can be rotated in the full erect position and the object deposited where desired.

Any rotation, however, is fraught with danger in that with the feet firmly planted on the ground, trunk twisting can injure the low back. Whenever possible, the feet should be *walked around* so that the object is lowered and deposited the proper way, namely, by deep knee bend, holding the object close to and in front of the body, and doing most of the work with a reasonably flat back and bent knees.

HABIT

The more that proper bending and re-extension are practiced, the more deeply ingrained they become. Habit now stands the patient in good stead. A person who is instructed and trained and who practices proper

146

bending, stooping, and re-extending to the erect position will do this automatically unless something unforeseen or unexpected intervenes. Providing training, practice, and repetition of proper lifting and bending is the purpose of a back school.

As previously stated, one of the most common causes of back pain is that, in spite of all the training, an unexpected distraction can cause the person at that very moment to bend, twist, lift, stoop, or squat in the wrong way. This distraction may be anger, impatience, haste, depression, tension, or other numerous interruptions and distractions.

The purpose of the Low Back School is to teach proper body movement in the hope that the patient will become so conditioned as not to allow or be caused to make faulty movements during periods of distraction.

WHEN IS LOW BACKACHE CONSIDERED CHRONIC?

A later chapter will be devoted to the treatment of chronic pain. The patient with chronic pain is one who continues to have pain lasting a long time that has failed to respond to usually effective, conservative treatment measures previously outlined. These are the persons with chronic back pain and chronic back disability who fail to respond to treatment and who do not regain comfort and function.

CONCLUSION

In this chapter, we have discussed treatment of acute low back pain and the cause and prevention of recurrent low back pain. It is apparent that all of the soft tissues of the functional unit must be considered in the treatment of low backache. These soft tissues include the muscles, the muscle fascial lining, the ligaments, the joint capsules, and tissues such as the cartilage of the joints, the disk, and the nerve roots contained within the functional unit. All must be considered.

CHAPTER 10

Surgery

INDICATIONS

Surgery is usually recommended when a patient has evidence of actual nerve damage or impending nerve damage that does not improve after a reasonable period of adequate conservative treatment. The patient now considered a surgical candidate shows objective evidence of nerve root damage. The feeling of numbness becomes definite loss of skin sensation. Weakness of the specific muscle groups that receive their nerve supply from that specific nerve root is now demonstrable.

Surgery is urgently considered when the patient exhibits loss of bowel or bladder function. There are special tests that can determine that the difficulty in voiding is caused by damage to the nerves going to the bowel or bladder and not from other unrelated causes.

SURGERY TO RELIEVE PAIN?

To operate merely to relieve pain is not, or should not be, an indication for surgery. Often patients complaining of persistent pain will influence the surgeon to consider surgical intervention in spite of minimal or no objective signs of nerve damage. Pain is so subjective, influenced by emotions, colored by secondary gains, and difficult to quantify objectively that surgical removal of pain cannot be expected, predicted, or certainly guaranteed. The potential undesirable sequelae of unsuccessful surgery, both physical and psychological, deter an experienced surgeon from rushing in for surgical intervention.

SURGERY: BY WHOM?

There is a conflict as to whether surgery should be performed by a neurosurgeon because nerves are involved, or by an orthopedic surgeon, because bone and joints are involved. Both may be competent depending on their training and the frequency with which they perform this procedure. Consultation and advice from a trusted family practitioner or primary physician may well influence the decision as to who will do the surgery. A university medical school or a medical society is always a good source of advice. Satisfactory results known to have occurred in many believable, reliable patients can be a good reference. Surgery performed in a reputable major hospital with high standards by a board-certified surgeon is the recommended course. Board certification and experience should be demanded from the surgeon consulted.

LAMINECTOMY OR LAMINOTOMY?

Removal of the offending tissue within the functional unit is the objective of surgery. This tissue that is pressing upon the nerve root, as a rule, is protruding disk material or a bone spur known as an osteophyte (Fig. 96).

Laminectomy or laminotomy is the surgical approach to seeing and ultimately removing the offending disk or osteophyte (see Fig. 96). *Laminotomy* implies removing a sufficient portion of the lamina to view the nerve within the neural canal or within the foramen. *Laminectomy* implies removing *all* that half of the lamina, thus giving a larger view of the disk and nerves or widening the neural canal to free the nerve root (Fig. 97).

Foraminotomy is a technique of widening a foramen that has been confirmed to be too narrow or deformed by a bone spur, thus being too narrow for the emerging nerve root. Before surgery, this narrow foramen is suspected then confirmed by visualizing it on oblique x-ray views, CAT scan, and/or a myelogram. Occasionally, the narrow foramen is visualized only by the surgeon during the operation.

Disk surgery is essentially *nuclectomy*. Actually, it is the nucleus that bulges or ruptures out of the disk that requires surgical removal. It is this portion of the disk that usually does the nerve damage. Surgery not only removes the bulging, ruptured portion of the nucleus with its pressure against the nerve but also intends to remove all of the remaining nucleus within the disk. Any part of the nucleus that would remain after surgery could ultimately rebulge or rerupture.

The annulus of the disk, which normally encircles and contains the nucleus, must have been torn to permit bulging or rupturing outward of the nucleus. Therefore, during surgery, this opening in the annulus must be made wider by the surgeon in order to remove the offending nucleus. If the nucleus has completely ruptured out of its containing annulus, it may be lying outside of the disk as a fragment within the neural canal. This fragment may be floating freely or may be trapped between the vertebral body and the nerve, thus placing the nerve under a great deal of tension.

149

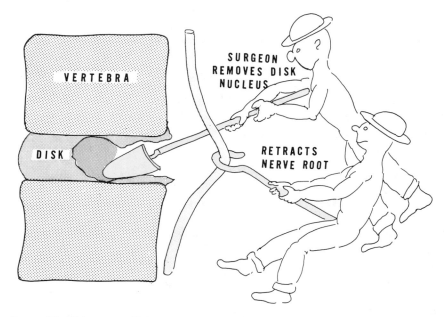

FIGURE 96. Disk surgery. This surgery is essentially removal of the nucleus (termed nuclectomy) and is often termed diskectomy. Laminotomy or laminectomy, part of this surgery, is discussed in the text and shown in Figure 97.

SPINAL FUSION

What Is It? What Is Done? Why Is It Done?

Initially, loss of the disk, either from rupture or from surgery, was believed to cause that particular functional unit to be unstable. Unstable was considered to imply collapse of one vertebra upon its adjacent vertebra within that functional unit. Excessive abnormal movement of the vertebral bodies could then be expected, since the vertebrae would no longer be kept apart by the normally expanded disk.

Weight bearing upon this functional unit without a functioning nucleus and disk would thus fall upon the facet joints, causing further gliding together. The foramen would obviously be narrowed and deformed.

Would Fusion Prevent This?

By fusion, new bone is placed between the facet joints and the lamina. The bone is gotten from cutting out the correct size and shape of a piece from the pelvis of the individual during the same operation. The facet

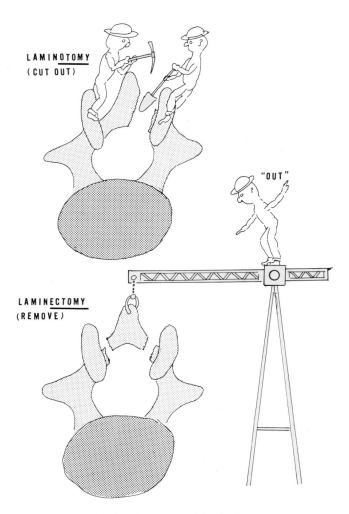

FIGURE 97. Laminectomy and laminotomy.

joints of the functional unit which are to be the receptor site of the fusion bone are prepared. The new fragment of bone is to be wedged in there. The receptor site is prepared by scraping off the cartilage of the facet joints. Eventually, the new piece of bone is placed and wedged between these two scraped bones. These merge into one bone, causing the functional unit to be fused.

Fusion has increasingly been considered of less value or benefit. It is rarely indicated. Only when excessive abnormal movement is shown to exist between two vertebrae and that abnormal movement has been de-

151

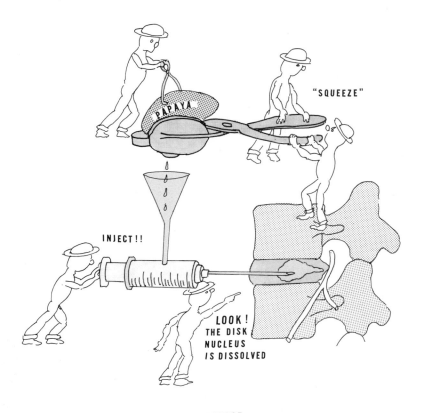

"SQUEEZE"

INJECT!!

LOOK!
THE DISK
NUCLEUS
IS DISSOLVED

CHYMOPAPASE

FIGURE 98. Nuclectomy by injection of chymopapase.

termined to produce pain or nerve damage is fusion considered to be indicated.

CHYMOPAPASE

A derivative of the Polynesian papaya fruit has been known to function as a meat tenderizer, or what is termed a proteolytic enzyme. *Proteo* means protein, and *lytic* means to dissolve. Papaya juice injected into an intervertebral disk dissolves the nucleus, which is protein (Fig. 98). Injection of papain into the nucleus does what is intended by surgery: it removes the nucleus.

Papaya has also been found to digest the annulus as well as the nucleus and thus narrow the disk space. Chymopapase, which is the term applied to papaya juice, was once considered capable of injuring the nerve sheath (coatings of the nerves) and the ligaments, so this procedure was not permitted in the United States. However, its value and safety have now been scientifically established, and its use has received approval by the FDA.

FAILED BACK SURGERY

This is a term currently used for unsuccessful surgery or for surgery to repair previous unsuccessful surgery—surgery apparently adequately performed after a clear indication for surgery that failed to accomplish its proper purpose, namely, relief of back pain, leg pain, numbness, and/or weakness. The reasons for surgical failure are multiple, but failure indicates a lack of complete knowledge of the many causes of low back pain and sciatic pain. Merely **cutting away what appears to be the offending tissue may not be the answer to successful treatment of disk disease.**

Pain is a subjective symptom that is not removable by a knife in spite of the enthusiasm of many surgeons. It is of interest that the number of back operations in the United States far exceeds those performed in European countries. It is also very interesting that in the United States there is a greater number of failed back surgeries.

Surgery too frequently adds new and different pains and impairment to those that existed prior to surgery, thus causing further reluctance of many patients and physicians today to consider surgical intervention.

It must always be remembered that it is a person being operated upon, not a back, a disk, an abnormal test, or a pain that has failed to respond to conservative nonsurgical treatment.

153

CHAPTER 11

Special Causes
of Low Back Pain

SPONDYLOLYSIS AND SPONDYLOLISTHESIS

Of the numerous mechanical causes of low back pain, there are two that deserve mention. These are spondylolysis and spondylolisthesis. The term *spondylo* means spine. The term *lysis* means a defect due to failure of bones to unite during their early formation. The term *listhesis* means slipping.

Spondylolysis

In early childhood, the bony arches that surround the dural canal, formed by the pedicles, the lamina, and the processors, are not completely formed into a complete ring. There are separate fragments of bone that gradually and ultimately join together, fusing into one continuous bone.

These bone fragments may fail to fuse at the region of the lamina, resulting in the defect that has been termed *lysis*. This defect may be on one side or on both sides. It may be present in one or both laminae. Lysis is seen frequently on x-ray but may be of no significance, not causing pain or disturbance.

Spondylolisthesis

If the lysis in the L4 or the L5 vertebral body bony structure permits definite separation, the uppermost vertebral body may slide forward upon the vertebra immediately below it. This sliding is permitted because the lysis defect has separated. This sliding of one vertebra upon the immediate inferior vertebra is termed *listhesis* (Fig. 99).

In listhesis, as the vertebra slide upon each other in an excessive or

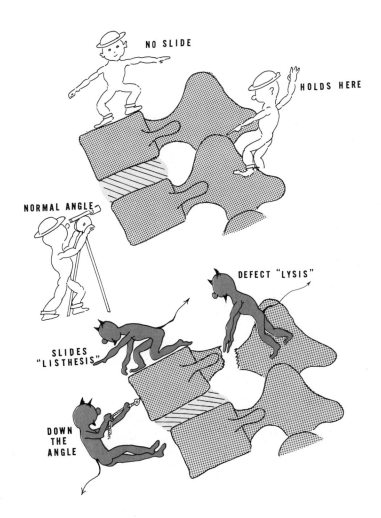

FIGURE 99. Spondylolysis and spondylolisthesis.

abnormal manner, shear is imposed on the disk that normally connects the two vertebral bodies together. This shear stress on the disk causes damage to the disk in that it stresses, strains, and tears the fibers of the annulus. Dehydration of the disk results as the fluid seeps out.

Not only does the disk space narrow, but the foramina, dependent upon an intact disk space, become deformed and narrowed. Pain in the low back can result from this disk narrowing due to the sliding forward of the vertebral bodies. Pain in the leg, or legs, can be felt from the foramen being deformed and its contained nerve roots being irritated.

155

A lysis defect is normally filled with fibrous tissue. This scarlike tissue either prevents sliding forward or at least prevents rapid or excessive sliding. A person can live a lifetime without pain or dysfunction from a lysis because the fibrous tissue may keep the bones together throughout life.

The fibrous tissue filling the lysis may be defective or injured, allowing separation and listhesis. Pain and/or impairment thus may result.

Treatment of Lysis and Listhesis

If there is bilateral lysis, the lower vertebra, which would allow forward sliding of the vertebra above due to its angulation, may be realigned to decrease the angle. The uppermost vertebra does not now have as acute an angle on which to slide. There is less tendency for the lysis to increase and for listhesis to result.

If listhesis occurs, progresses, and becomes symptomatic, surgery may be necessary. The purpose of surgery in this situation is to fuse the lysis surgically to prevent further listhesis. Unfortunately, repair of the listhesis rarely corrects the degree of forward sliding; it merely stops further sliding at that point.

In addition to fusing of the lysis, it is possible to remove the remaining fragments of bones behind the lysis that may be causing pain.

CANCER

Cancer is considered to be one of the more ominous causes of low back pain. Cancer may be primary or secondary. Primary cancer is cancer of the bone that begins in the bone and resides within the bone itself until it spreads to the surrounding areas.

This type of cancer causes pain that is insidious in that it is constant or nocturnal. It is felt at night, frequently keeping the patient awake. It is, as a rule, not related to movement, to position, or to activity. These two factors—(1) constant pain, primarily at night and (2) pain not related to movement or activity—are clues to the physician that the problem is not mechanical but is within the bones.

There are other signs frequently associated with cancer, such as weight loss, fatigue, and loss of appetite. If the cancer has spread, it will cause symptoms in the organs into which it spreads.

Cancer of the bone is frequently first noted on routine x-ray and later in nuclear scans and in CAT scans. Treatment depends on the type of tissue of the cancer, whether cancer is primary or metastatic, and at which stage it is.

ARTHRITIS

The term arthritis is unfortunately frequently misused, overused, or abused as the diagnosis of the cause of back pain.

In the acute inflammatory arthritis of the rheumatoid variant, the most frequent is the Marie-Strumpell rheumatoid spondylitis. This is rheumatoid arthritis of the spine, hence the term spondylitis. It is known also as ankylosing spondylitis. The term ankylosing means hardening and stiffening. This inflammatory disease of the spine causes the condition termed bamboo spine.

Ankylosing spondylitis is a disease occurring 10 times more often in males than in females and frequently in members of the same family. This condition, occurring in a young male in late adolescence or his early 20s, starts with low back discomfort described as stiffness or aching, usually noted in the morning. At first, the discomfort generally is so insignificant that the patient does not go to a physician. As time passes, however, the severity, limitation, and stiffness increase.

The diagnosis is suggested in a young male complaining of early morning stiffness and increasing stiffness with activity. Gradually x-rays show a hardening or an obliteration of the sacroiliac joints. These are the joints found between the ilium and the sacrum, as was shown in Chapter 1. In patients with ankylosing spondylitis, this joint at first appears hazy and fuzzy and eventually solidifies and becomes fused. The ligaments that run the entire length of the spine gradually become calcified. The bones undergo decalcification (osteoporosis), giving the appearance of bamboo on x-ray. There are special blood tests that aid in confirming the diagnosis of ankylosing spondylitis.

The unfortunate aspect of this disease at this time is that although the pain and discomfort can be alleviated with exercises and medicine, the disease process continues with subsequent stiffening. The intent of treatment is to have the spine stiffen in a functional and cosmetically acceptable way from neck to sacrum.

RHEUMATOID ARTHRITIS

Rheumatoid arthritis, in contrast to ankylosing spondylitis, strikes women three times more often than men. Rheumatoid arthritis is inflammatory and usually affects peripheral joints such as hands, elbows, feet, toes, knees, and other joints of the body before the spine itself becomes involved. The spine, however, is also subject to inflammatory changes but does not necessarily undergo the same type of bamboo sclerosing as does Marie-Strumpell spondylitis.

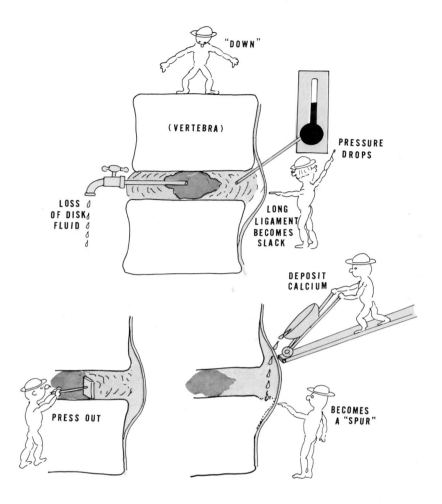

FIGURE 100. Formation of an "osteophyte:" degenerative arthritis.

DEGENERATIVE ARTHRITIS:
OSTEOARTHRITIS VERSES OSTEOARTHROSIS

There are numerous labels for the process of degenerative arthritis; osteoarthritis is the most commonly used. Osteoarthritis is extremely common. It is as old as antiquity, having been observed in skeletons of Neanderthal man 40,000 B.C.

Even the term osteoarth*ritis* is a misnomer, since this is not an inflammatory disease as the suffix *itis* indicates. Degenerative arthritis is basi-

158

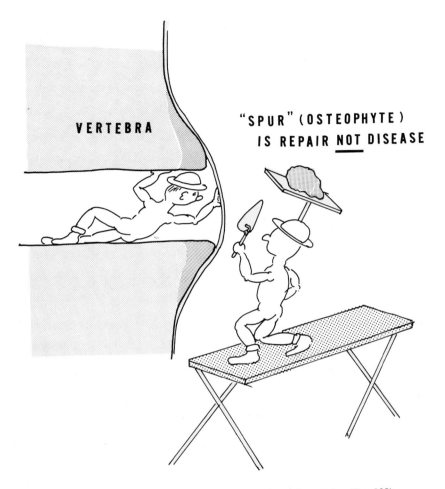

VERTEBRA

"SPUR" (OSTEOPHYTE)
IS REPAIR **NOT** DISEASE

FIGURE 101. More on the formation of an arthritic "spur" (see Fig. 100).

cally osteoarth*rosis*, indicating a process of wear and tear, repaired by nature with the formation of bone.

This is a disease process of movable, **weight bearing** joints with progressive degeneration of cartilage. In the case of the lumbar spine, it is the intervertebral disk that degenerates first, then the facets. The progressive changes in these joints consist of laying down of bone beneath the cartilage to repair the damaged cartilage.

This disease process is more commonly found in the elderly and is considered an inherent part of the aging process. There are no micro-

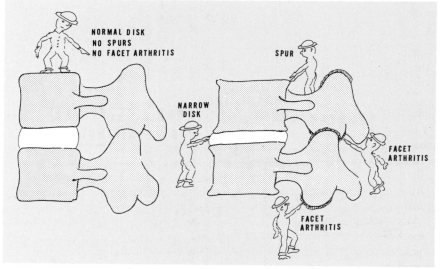

FIGURE 102. Degenerative arthritis of the facet joints secondary to disk degeneration (narrowing).

scopic changes in arthritic cartilage that differ from normal aging processes. Other factors contribute to the appearance, rapidity, and development of osteoarthrosis. These factors are compression, injury, excessive use, and congenital predisposition.

Degenerative disease of the spine affects two joints of the functional unit: the disk and the facet joints. The disk initiates the process. Annular fibers are repeatedly damaged. The nucleus leaks out and dehydrates (dries up). This process decreases the pressure within the disk, allowing the vertebral bodies to come closer together.

The long ligaments become slack as the result of the vertebrae reapproaching. These long ligaments pull away from their attachments to the vertebrae. The disk material, still under pressure, squeezes out between the vertebrae and the ligament, further peeling away the ligament (Fig. 100).

This protruding of disk material occurs slowly over a long period of time. With the seepage from the area of irritated bone where the ligament has peeled away, a hardened mass of tissues forms, which ultimately becomes calcified. Calcified means deposit of calcium that forms bone. This calcified mass forms a spur, termed osteophyte (Fig. 101).

X-rays of osteoarthrosis reveals the narrowed joint space where the degenerated disk is. The spurs can be noted on each side, front and back, of the vertebral column.

The other joints of the functional unit, the facets, also undergo degenerative changes. They have cartilage of the two surfaces that face each other. Normally, the facets do not bear weight but merely glide on each other. If the disk up front allows the vertebrae to approximate, the facets also approximate and become weight bearing. Now, as they glide during any movement, they wear away the degenerated cartilage (Fig. 102).

The cartilage of the facet joints goes through the same changes as do joints throughout the body. The cartilage wears, the joint narrows, bone is laid down in the damaged cartilage-bone area, and osteophytes form there.

Symptoms are pain on weight bearing, stiffness after periods of immobilization, aching when fatigued, and limited movement. If the osteophytes are large enough, they can encroach upon the nerve within the foramen, causing nerve symptoms.

With spurs formed anteriorly at the disk level and posteriorly from the facets, the foramen can be markedly narrowed. With the long ligaments slack, even though irritated and thickened, the functional unit can have abnormal movement. Pain can result.

Treatment aims to maintain good posture and good flexibility. Weight bearing is an important factor; therefore, weight loss is mandatory. All instructions regarding proper bending and lifting are also indicated.

It is of interest and significance that this type of arthritis responds well to the salicylates. Aspirin derivatives are the most important form of drug that can be given to the patient with degenerative arthritis.

It is unfortunate that many patients are labeled as suffering from degenerative arthritis as *the cause* of their back pain, when essentially one of the other mechanical factors imposed upon the degenerated spine is causing their pain. Hence, to label a patient as having backache from degenerative arthritis until other mechanical causes have been established is a disfavor to the patient and one that is fraught with failure unless mechanically corrected.

CHAPTER 12

Psychological Aspects
of Low Back Pain

The term *psychological* is applied to any disease, impairment, disability, or painful condition of mankind that is afflicted, aggravated, intensified, or initiated by the emotions.

There is no disease that does not have an emotional component that causes, aggravates, or intensifies the symptoms by its presence.

For centuries, patients have had psychosomatic illness. *Psycho* means the psychological aspects; *somatic* means the tissue changes that a person undergoes when an illness or impairment is sustained as a result of emotional trauma. The relationship of the psyche and the soma has been predominant in recent centuries of medical care.

Unfortunately, this concept often has been overemphasized, misapplied, frequently misconceived, and therefore misconstrued. The patient has been almost universally accused rather than diagnosed by this label as having an imaginary illness. This may be true in a slight percentage of patients but is not necessarily true in most.

There is no doubt that the emotions play a very large part in the causation of painful conditions such as low back pain. The low back does not function well when a person is upset, angry, irate, impatient, or depressed. As was stated in previous chapters, the entire mechanism of function and the precisely skilled musculoskeletal control are impaired when a person's psychological picture is upset.

Pain is always felt more strongly in an emotionally upset individual. A headache in a woman whose marriage is unhappy will be more severe than a headache in someone who is otherwise emotionally at peace with the world and with herself. Psychological studies have verified that pain is intensified in a person who is under emotional duress.

Consequently, there is every evidence that low back pain is markedly aggravated, more prevalent, more prominent, and more resistant to treatment in a person who is emotionally distraught than it would be in a person who is emotionally calm, under good control, or at peace with himself.

SECONDARY GAINS

The concept of secondary gains has also suffered from misinterpretation. Secondary gains have been attributed to the fact that by having back symptoms a person can get monetary reward or be excused from participating in what is otherwise a threatening or an unpleasant situation or occupation. No doubt secondary financial gains play a factor in persistent disability. The industrially injured patient is a good example of this type of secondary gain, as is the patient suffering from a personal injury.

The industrially injured patient may not particularly enjoy working with the particular supervisor. The person on a job who does not enjoy the circumstances of that work or the remuneration from that work may feel justification in not reporting for work by virtue of back symptoms. This is a secondary gain that may be conscious, but in many cases it is subconscious or even totally unconscious.

An example of secondary gains is the fright of the person who has sustained an injury from an auto accident, an altercation with a belligerent individual, or an altercation of a frightening nature. The incident may have caused pain that is not diagnosed or diagnosable. The fear of what this back pain may mean may cause this person to have symptoms far exceeding actual organic damage.

Secondary gains also have some psychological value. There is no doubt that a person who cannot perform a specific activity by virtue of low back pain is essentially having secondary gain. This secondary gain need not be financial, but it may be a reward justified by the symptom of low back pain.

The physician is placed in a position of judgment in accepting and justifying that the person's low back pain prevents performance of the occupation or activity. The physician is omnipotent in this respect. The judgment of disabling low back pain is frequently made by the physician at the subconscious request of the patient. Frequently this is misused, and occasionally it is abused. This is, however, the situation as it exists in the 20th century and will undoubtedly continue for decades to come.

Low back pain is sanctioned as a cause for a person to receive insurance payments, industrial indemnity remuneration, or a judgment from personal injury cases. Verification is usually based on the statement of the physician.

163

TERTIARY GAINS

Tertiary gains is a recent psychological term that asserts that a third party may benefit from a second party being disabled. The second party essentially has the secondary gains.

An example of tertiary gain is the wife of a man who is injured at work in an area in which she, the wife, does not wish to live or in an occupation in which she does not wish to have her husband employed. By virtue of the injury and its disability, the husband is compensated and excused from working. By virtue of the low back disability, the husband becomes vocationally retrained, which permits a change geographically as well as a change in the type of job. The wife in this case receives tertiary gains. This is merely one of many examples of tertiary gain.

DIAGNOSIS OF PSYCHOLOGICAL APPROACHES

In the past, professors of psychiatry believed that there was such an individual as a pain-prone patient. These people are characterized as being more susceptible to injury with resultant pain. Low back pain is a predominant site of pain. These pain-prone people were characterized as being unhappy or in need of pain for self-punishment. They received attention or relief of their guilt feelings through the pain that they were feeling.

Pain-prone people may well exist, although this has not yet been well accepted or standardized. There are psychiatrically ill people in whom pain is a symptom. This symptom can be treated after it has been recognized by a psychiatrist.

It is extremely difficult to make a diagnosis of pain-proneness as a psychological abnormality, although one may be suspicious when an individual sustains painful injuries or has accidents more frequently or repeatedly than can be considered average. Excessive symptomatology for minor organic abnormalities is also a clue in the frequently injured person.

Figure Drawings

A test is frequently given by doctors or psychologists to determine whether the symptoms are organic or highly imaginary. A drawing of a person is given to the patient (Fig. 103) to identify the site *where* the pain is felt and *what* sensation is felt. Sites drawn that cannot be anatomically or neurologically feasible will arouse suspicion that there is a strong emotional component.

The character of the pain also colors the deduction of the examiner as to the symptoms being bizarre or exaggerated. Malingerers will distort this test but the test *does not* differentiate between overreaction on an emotional basis and malingering.

164

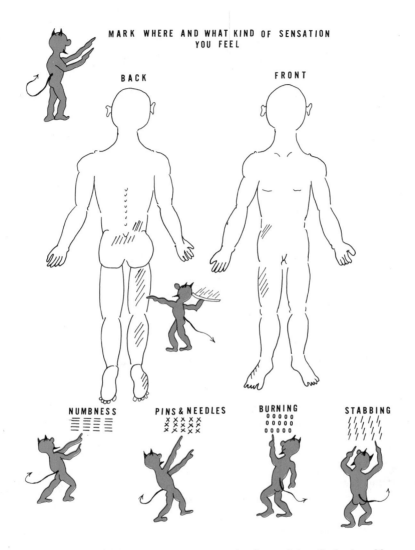

FIGURE 103. "Sensory map" designed by patient to localize and describe back and leg symptoms.

M.M.P.I.: What Is It?

Numerous tests are considered valid in differentiating the psychological aspects of pain. The test that has been used most frequently and upon which physicians and psychologists rely is the Minnesota Multiphasic Personality Inventory (M.M.P.I.).

165

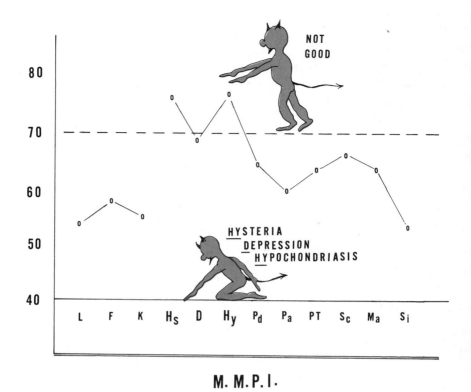

FIGURE 104. Minnesota Multiphasic Personality Inventory (M.M.P.I.)

The M.M.P.I. is one of the most researched instruments in psychological testing. It is an objective test to ascertain the presence of psychopathology (psychological disease or abnormality) or personality disorder.

The M.M.P.I. consists of 566 true or false statements that the patient is asked to answer during a limited period of time. The statements relate to attitudes, past behaviors, preferences, sensations, and experience.

The answers have been standardized and allow the interpreter to scale numerically and code the answers according to various categories. These scales measure the presence of personality disorders or psychiatric defects such as hypochondriasis, depression, hysteria, psychopathic deviation, sexual deviation, psychasthenia, schizophrenia, mania, paranoia, and social introversion. The interpretation is not based solely on the analysis of one of the scales but rather on the configuration of the entire M.M.P.I. profile (Fig. 104).

166

Built into the test is a group of scales called validity scales that enable the interpreter of the M.M.P.I. to ascertain whether or not the person taking the test is purposely or intentionally feigning psychiatric illness or intentionally attempting to deny psychiatric illness.

In patients with chronic pain, the M.M.P.I. frequently shows an elevation of hysteria, hypochondriasis, and depression. The M.M.P.I. is undergoing intensive use and an increasing amount of interpretation. As recently as 1982, it has been determined that the M.M.P.I. does not differentiate between pain from chronic illness and chronic pain with no organic component. It has not been determined whether the elevation of these three M.M.P.I. scales occurs when pain is of a chronic nature that has persisted rather than when pain persists and becomes chronic because of the personality impairment. There is no doubt that depression, hysteria, and hypochondriasis can intensify the sensation of pain and even cause pain to become chronic.

The M.M.P.I., however, remains a valid test, but it must be used carefully as a supplementary test and as confirmation of a clinically suspected psychologically afflicted patient. It cannot per se label a patient as psychologically influencing the severity of pain.

CHAPTER 13

Chronic Low Back Pain

WHEN DOES ACUTE PAIN BECOME CHRONIC PAIN?

As compared with acute pain, chronic pain is arbitrarily defined as pain that has persisted for 6 months or longer and has persisted in spite of every known accepted and applied treatment. Chronic pain also implies impairment far exceeding what could be expected from the discernible abnormalities. Chronic pain can also be viewed as disability (inability to function) far exceeding impairment (structural changes preventing function).

The examination of a patient with chronic low back pain must review and evaluate every potential cause of pain. This must be done to justify the term chronic pain.

A more recent definition of chronic pain is pain that is now central, not needing any irritating stimuli approaching the central nervous system from the periphery.

What this means in nonmedical terminology is that the pain is felt in the brain by virtue of a reverberating circuit in the spinal cord. There is no longer a need of its being fed irritating impulses from the disk, the ligaments, the muscles, the joints, or the tendons of the spine or the extremity.

A person who has chronic pain of this type feels pain but not because the brain is still being fed irritating input from the tissues of the spine or its vicinity. All tests of the spine such as x-rays, E.M.G.s, and nuclear scans are now essentially unrevealing. Movements of a specific nature no longer specifically aggravate the pain. Conservative management such as exercise and medication is no longer beneficial.

Examination of the person with chronic pain thus essentially becomes examination *of the person,* not of the pain and its mechanisms. It implies learning about the *meaning of pain to the patient and what pain allows or prevents that person's function to be.*

Secondary Gains

Secondary gains become meaningful in that there may be reward in painful disability. A frightening or threatening situation may be avoided, as may a failure or overwhelming stress, by the patient complaining of pain.

Malingering

Secondary gain may be financial or psychological. In most cases, this gain is unconscious or subconscious. Conscious or willful secondary gain may be considered *malingering*, which is probably more infrequent than currently suspected. Malingering is essentially an accusation rather than a diagnosis; whereas psychologically unconscious secondary gain is a diagnosis that justifies treatment. Both do exist and can be established to exist, albeit with trepidation by the physician.

TREATMENT IS DIFFICULT

Treatment of chronic pain is intended to permit the patient to function. The patient is trained to cope with a pain that may be only modified but not eliminated. Treatment of chronic pain, so labeled and defined, is thus psychological. Modalities are used that attempt to modify the pain to a tolerable level.

WHAT IS A MODALITY?

A modality is a treatment, physical or otherwise, applied to a patient that will benefit the patient by diminishing the sensation of pain, decreasing the severity of pain, or reducing the anxiety or fear of the pain.

TENS

TENS, abbreviation for *transcutaneous electrical nerve stimulation*, is the application of electrical current of specific form, shape, and frequency. It is applied by means of electrodes attached to the skin. The applied current travels via a nerve root to the central nervous system to diminish the transmitted pain-producing input in that nerve. Theoretically, there are two different impulses that travel along the nerve at different speeds. The electrical nerve stimulation (TENS), to be effective, must be varied to each individual and be applied at different sites along the nerve. The current must be varied at different wave frequencies, form sequences, and in duration. The instruments that deliver these currents allow these adjustments but must be varied for each patient. Some patients happily get excellent results. Some get benefit for a brief period, and unfortunately, some receive no relief. There is no way other than by trial to determine who will benefit and to what extent.

BIOFEEDBACK

Biofeedback is self-training of the individual to influence the sensation and bodily reaction that were previously considered autonomic, and thus not under voluntary control.

These autonomic bodily reactions include pulse rate, blood pressure, body temperature, and perspiration. These are functions of the autonomic nervous system. The other nervous system is termed the somatic nervous system, which is the nervous system under the person's voluntary control. The somatic nervous system permits voluntary contraction of muscle, thus permitting function such as manual actions, walking, running, and even the voluntary muscular reaction of taking a deep breath. The autonomic nervous system reacts reflexively with little or no control by the person.

Biofeedback training may be performed by eliciting noises, sounds, visual images, or electrical impulse responses to bodily functions. The ancient yogis of India developed these controls without instruments.

IMAGERY

Imagery is a form of self-hypnosis in which a pleasant image can be conjured, or self-imposed, by the person to replace a threatening or unpleasant situation. The afflicted person develops a serene, relaxed, pleasant scene of situation or environment. By so doing, the environment that has been related to the sensation of pain or influenced by the pain is removed or improved.

PROGRESSIVE RELAXATION

A muscle, or group of muscles, can normally be caused to contract. A tense muscle may, however, be contracted without voluntary control. A muscle voluntarily contracted normally can be voluntarily relaxed, whereas a tense muscle, not under voluntary control, cannot be voluntarily relaxed.

Sustained muscle tension becomes painful. This pain can be relieved or diminished if the muscle can be relaxed.

In progressive relaxation, a person is trained to voluntarily contract a muscle, then trained to voluntarily relax the muscle. Relaxing a muscle that is or has been painful results in less pain and in greater movement and function.

DRUGS

Most patients with chronic pain become dependent on drugs. The symptoms do not usually respond to drugs, thus the patient becomes addicted to drugs of limited value in search of pain relief. Much of the treatment for chronic pain attempts to eliminate or minimize this drug dependency.

Anti-inflammatory Drugs

The value of some drugs is based on the assumption that pain may be due partly to tissue inflammation. These anti-inflammatory drugs have become accepted for their value. These anti-inflammatory drugs are as-pirinlike in their action.

Non-narcotic pain medications, or pain-relieving drugs, also exist, but these unfortunately do not retain their efficacy and may lead to increasing and excessive use, dependency, or a transfer to stronger drugs.

Drugs to Allay Depression

Antidepressant drugs have proven to be of great value. Many patients suffering from chronic pain have an underlying depression that may benefit from antidepressant drugs. Recently, there has been evidence that some antidepressant drugs also stimulate the normal, bodily created pain-modifying enzymes of the individual. These enzymes have been called endorphins.

ACUPUNCTURE

Acupuncture involves the insertion of needles into the body at specific locations. For centuries in oriental cultures, acupuncture has enjoyed acceptance as being curative for numerous diseases and very beneficial in the relief of pain. It has also been found to be valuable in the induction of anesthesia, which is in essence elimination of sensation as well as minimization of the perception of pain.

Its value in North America is under study, but acupuncture is not yet a generally accepted concept or technique. Acupuncture may not necessarily be beneficial, but it is not considered harmful, except as an added financial burden to an already financially overburdened patient (Fig. 105).

171

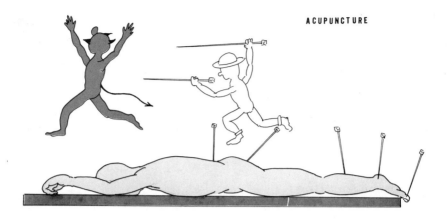

FIGURE 105. Acupuncture.

PSYCHOTHERAPY

Assuming that the treatment of chronic pain is the psychological reorientation of the patient, psychotherapy is the fundamental basis of most treatment programs. There are numerous forms of psychological help, all with their fervent advocates.

Counseling, group therapy, analysis, and operant conditioning are some of the accepted therapeutic approaches. A competent, trained, and interested psychiatrist or psychologist is best qualified to evaluate the patient. The significance of psychological factors in the chronic pain patient and the patient's potential response to psychological intervention require careful testing and interview.

Acceptance of psychological influence of chronic pain by the patient is mandatory before benefit from psychotherapy can be expected. Denial of possible psychological aspects to pain eliminates any possible benefit from this type of treatment.

It must never be stated that pain is all in the mind. This implies an imaginary cause of pain and denies that physical pain can be seriously influenced by the emotions. The meaning of pain must be clarified. There is a fine line as to whether chronic pain results in an emotional reaction or whether the emotions instigate the chronicity of pain. Both aspects undoubtedly contribute and thus both must be considered.

172

Epilogue

In the final analysis, what is the bottom line as to *the* cause of most low backaches? The question relates to the mechanical low backaches, not to those from malignancy, fracture, or infection where the cause is more obvious.

It must be stated emphatically that there is *no one* cause and effect of low backache that is universally accepted. There are numerous causes claimed for low backache, so to claim *the* cause is merely to express one's personal opinion.

Is there a common denominator to many low backaches? Is there an explanation of WHY, WHERE, and HOW low back pain occurs? If there is a common denominator, does it justify the numerous tests and forms of treatment advocated for low back pain? A YES answer, whether strong or weak, must justify the proposed explanation.

In this book, functional anatomy has received a great deal of emphasis. The spine is a functional unit that operates on mechanical principles. To know these is to know HOW the spine works. It is important to know HOW the spine functionally is injured, misused, or impaired to understand WHY and HOW low back pain can occur.

In review of the anatomical structure of the lumbar spine, the *functional unit* has been designated as to WHERE pain can occur. This functional unit consists of two vertebrae separated by a hydraulic disk. There are numerous tissues within the unit that when irritated can cause pain, but it is the *disk* that absorbs the numerous shocks to the spine. The disk permits the spine to bend, twist, extend, and lift. The disk is obviously a very important piece of tissue within the unit that determines how the functional unit, and hence the entire vertebral column, functions or malfunctions.

How does the disk function, how does it get injured, and how does it repair itself? These are questions that need to be answered. How does injury to the disk and to the functional unit as a result of disk injury result

173

in pain and disability? With this answer, the basis for treatment and, more important, how to prevent reinjury can be stated.

Merely discussing disk injury as *the* cause of low back pain would be simplistic and a mistake, as the disk is not the *only* cause of low back pain. It may not be *the* cause, but it certainly may contribute to the cause of pain. Insult to one of the many painful tissues within the functional unit must be the cause of pain, with the disk in some way being responsible for that tissue injury. This is a more plausible answer.

The disk is chemically and structurally similar to cartilage anywhere in the body. It is largely water (88 percent) and acts like a sponge. When squeezed, fluid seeps out. When pressure is released, fluid is absorbed *back into* the disk (sponge). This fluid absorbed into the sponge is its nutrition. To remain viable and functional, cartilage must be *repeatedly squeezed* but especially *released*. It is during release of pressure that nutrition enters the tissue.

The tissue structure that contains the fluid is the annulus. The annulus is made of fibers that attach from one vertebra to the adjacent vertebra. They crisscross each other, lending strength to the disk. These fibers stretch very little and are kept taut by the pressure within the disk nucleus, which is in the center completely encircled by the annulus. The internal nuclear pressure keeps the vertebrae apart.

The structural unit is held in good balance by the integrity of all these tissues: the nucleus, the annulus, and the long ligaments. If the annular fibers are torn, fluid leaks out. The vertebrae come closer together and the long ligaments become slack. The bony structures behind the vertebrae, such as the pedicles and the facets, come closer together. The foramen narrows, thus compressing the nerve roots contained therein. The facet joints lose their proper alignment.

Inflammation of all these disrupted tissues causes the muscles to go into spasm to prevent further movement and possible further tissue inflammation. This spasm itself can become a source of pain. Prolonged or repeated muscle spasm causes the muscles to shorten. Movement of the spine becomes limited. The cycle is evident.

What can initiate this cycle that ends in low backache?

There are several factors that predominate:

In an emotionally tense person, whether this is an acute or chronic condition, the muscles of the body, including the low back muscles, never completely relax. During sustained muscular contraction of the spine, the disk also is never relaxed, and thus never can imbibe its nutritive fluid. The disk also does not intermittently squeeze out its unwanted tissue substances that accumulate from a compressed disk tissue. Disk degeneration results, initiating a sequence of changes.

The low back muscles, not relaxing, cannot lengthen. Without relaxation and elongation of the back muscles, the low back cannot flex. Once

174

flexed to its slight degree, the back does not properly re-extend to the erect posture, since a tense muscle does not smoothly shorten any more than it can lengthen. Any intended or needed movement such as sitting, bending, stooping, or lifting now is done improperly, erratically, and painfully. This improper movement due to muscle tension may injure the tissues of the functional unit, resulting in pain.

A poorly conditioned individual may move properly, but the tissues of the spine cannot accomplish the needed movement, so injuries result.

Which tissue or tissues within the functional unit are injured, resulting in pain? The limitation of movement and the movement or position that causes the pain indicate WHERE pain occurs.

Improper sway back posture places weight upon the sensitive facet joints that normally should not bear significant weight. This posture also causes the foramen to narrow, thus compressing the nerve within the foramen. Leg pain, leg weakness, or leg numbness results along the distribution of the nerve root.

A rupture of the disk pressing directly upon the posterior long ligament can result in limited forward flexion of the spine with low back ache. The pain in the low back becomes aggravated by flexing the neck after the back has been flexed as much as the patient can tolerate. This movement increases the tension on the long ligament. The pain that results is attributable to long ligament irritation due to central disk herniation.

If a disk herniates (ruptures) to one side, it can press on the nerve root passing by the disk on that side and at that vertebral level. There are tests such as straight leg raising, checking reflexes, and testing sensation or muscle strength that confirm this possibility.

In essence, there are movements done by the patient or by the physician that specify which tissue to incriminate as causing the pain in or from the low back.

Tests, be they x-rays, myelogram, CAT scans, or E.M.G., merely confirm what a careful clinical examination reveals or implies. These tests must *always* be related to the results of the examination and not be interpreted in isolation.

An excessively strenuous or unexpectedly light activity that occurs when the person is unprepared for that action can injure the back even if the activity is within the capabilities of that person and the person is in good mental and physical condition. The effort is not consistent or appropriate for that task. Too much or too little effort and movement result. Tissues are strained and injured.

A stress imposed upon the person who is not expecting it due to tension, anger, fatigue, or depression may also *catch* the body unprepared.

Whatever the initiating reason for the improper movement or position, the result is the same. There is tissue injury with resultant inflammation, causing spasm, limitation, and pain.

The diagnosis is based upon *what* happened and *when* and *how* it happened. Detailing the exact movement or position of the body at the time of injury specifies the *how*.

Treatment begins with rest of the injured tissues early to initiate repair and decrease of inflammation. Rest is accomplished by body position, drugs, other modalities, and time. Reconditioning the tissues follows by means of exercises to improve flexibility and strength. Retraining the individual on the care and proper use of the back follows.

When spinal malalignment exists, it needs to be discovered and corrected. When tissue damage has been significant, causing damage to nerve tissues, it may need to be removed by surgical means.

If the person has a controlling emotional problem that adversely influences proper activities or intensifies the resultant symptoms and pain, this has to be recognized and treated.

There may be greater duration of disabling pain than expected for the severity of the injury or the resultant tissue damage. If the pain does not respond to time and adequate treatment, the *person*, not the backache, must now receive the attention.

Glossary

Acupressure. Pressure on any part of the body to decrease pain without use of needles.

Acupuncture. Insertion of needles into certain parts of the body to decrease pain. Considered to stimulate endorphins.

Ankle reflex. Also called ankle jerk. A reflex of the ankle when Achilles tendon is tapped with reflex hammer. Implies reaction of the S_1 nerve root. Is called present, diminished, or absent.

Annulus fibrosus. The ringlike fibrous tissue of the invertebral disk surrounding the nucleus, connecting the vertebral bodies, crisscrossed for strength.

Biofeedback. Attempts to train a person to develop control of functions of the body under autonomic control such as temperature, pulse, and blood pressure. Also used to control anxiety and tension due to emotions.

Bowstring test. With patients who have sciatica, pressure behind the bent knee upon the nerve roots causes pain.

Bragard's test. During straight leg raising, dorsiflexion of the foot causes pain along the course of the sciatic nerve. Indicates the nerve dura is inflamed.

Bulging disk. Herniation or protrusion of the annulus of the disk outside of the normal confines.

Cartilage. A specialized connective tissue. A tissue that lines the ends of bones of most joints. Lines the facet joints of the spine.

CAT scan. Abbreviation for computerized axial tomography. Specialized x-ray technique that reveals three planes of bones, joints, and organs. Reveals soft tissues as well as bones. Also called CT scan.

Cauda equina. The nerves that become divided from the spinal cord at the thoracolumbar junction to form nerve roots. Cauda equina means horse's tail in Latin.

Cervical spine. The seven vertebrae in the neck region.

177

Chymopapase. An enzyme derived from a tropical fruit, papaya. It is currently used to dissolve disks chemically rather than remove them surgically. Also called papase.

Coccyx. The lower end of the spinal column; the few small bones forming the tail.

Cortisone. A hormone secreted by the adrenal glands, now also chemically manufactured. It combats inflammation.

Degenerated disk. Deterioration of the substance of the disk; causes include dehydration, fibrosis, and shrinking.

Dehydration. Loss of water content.

Dermatome. An area of the skin supplied by a specific nerve root.

Disc versus disk. The word with "c" or "k" indicates the same tissue spelled differently; both spellings are accepted.

Disk. A water-containing gelatinous mass (mucopolysaccharide) surrounded by circumferential fibers, between two vertebrae; acts to cushion the functional unit and permit spinal flexibility.

Diskectomy. Removal of the disk either surgically or chemically. A treatment for a damaged disk that causes symptoms.

Diskitis. Inflammation of a disk. The ending "itis" indicates inflammation.

Diskogram. An x-ray picture of the disk nucleus after a dye has been injected. A test to determine disk rupture or degeneration and specify which disk.

Dura. Fibrous "skin" that forms sheath or sleeve around the nerve roots.

Endorphins. Morphinelike substance allegedly generated by the body to combat pain.

Excised disk. A disk that has been completely or partially removed.

Extruded disk. A term alternately used with ruptured or protruded disk, i.e., one that has been forced out of its normal position between two adjacent vertebrae.

Facet. Joints behind the vertebral bodies that glide on each other, allowing movement in flexion and extension, and preventing side movement and rotation.

Facetectomy. Surgical removal of the facet joint.

Foramen. The opening between two adjacent vertebrae of the spinal column at each functional unit through which the nerve roots pass.

Fragmented disk. A term used by some to mean ruptured disk.

Functional impairment. Although this term designates function, it is used to imply psychological rather than organic impairment.

Functional unit. Arbitrary designation of two adjacent vertebrae and the interposed disk with all the included tissues.

Hernia. Protrusion of tissue through an abnormal opening.

Herniated disk. Similar to bulging or ruptured disk. Means that disk material, either nucleus or annulus of a disk, has left its normal confines.

Immobilization. Prevention of movement or activity.

Intervertebral. Between two vertebrae.

Intervertebral disk. The fibrocartilaginous disk between two adjacent vertebrae, which form a functional unit.

Iliac bone. Bilateral bones forming the pelvis, connected behind to the sacrum.

Knee jerk. The reflex elicited by striking the patellar tendon below the knee.

Knee reflex. The proper medical term for the knee jerk. Tests the femoral nerve, or the nerve roots L_2-L_3.

Kyphosis. The curvature of the thoracic spine with posterior convexity.

Lamina. The flattened part of either side of the arch of a vertebra.

Laminectomy. Surgical removal of a portion of the lamina. This procedure exposes the nerve roots and the disk in spinal surgery.

Laminotomy. Removal of only a small segment of the lamina (see text).

Lasegue test. Another name for the straight leg raising test.

Ligament. A band of connective tissue: dense, white, fibrous tissue that connects adjacent bony protrusions to stabilize a joint or limit movement.

Longitudinal ligament. A wide, long ligament that lines the vertebral bodies. These also constitute the outer layer of the annulus. There is a ligament down the front of the vertebra termed the anterior longitudinal ligament and one down the rear portion of the vertebra termed the posterior longitudinal ligament.

Lordosis. The curve formed in the cervical and lumbar spine. Concavity is behind.

Lumbar spine. The five vertebrae below the thoracic spine and above the sacrum.

Lumbar puncture. Entry into the dural sheath by a long needle to withdraw spinal fluid or inject the myelogram dye.

Metrizamide. A water-soluble dye injected into the dura to perform a myelogram.

Myelogram. A dye test to determine the presence and the site of a herniated disk or a tumor within the dural space of the spinal canal.

Myotome. The specific muscle or muscles that are stimulated to contract via one nerve root.

Mucopolysaccharide. A complex protein that is found in the disk material.

Nerve root. A nerve fiber that originates from the spinal cord and leaves the spinal column through the foramen.

Neurologist. A physician who specializes in diagnosing and treating diseases of the nervous system.

179

Neurosurgeon. A physician, a surgeon, specializing in diseases of the nervous system amenable to surgical removal.

Nucleus. The central gelatinous core of any complex that serves a specific function.

Nucleus pulposus. The central pulp mass of the disk held in the center of the encircling annular fibers. It is under intrinsic pressure and keeps the vertebrae apart.

Orthopedist. A physician who specializes in diseases of the musculoskeletal system.

Pantopaque. An insoluble dye injected into the dura for performing a myelogram. Unlike metrizamide, it is *not* water-soluble and must be withdrawn after the test.

Papase. An enzyme derived from a tropical fruit, papaya. It is currently used to dissolve disks chemically rather than remove them surgically. Also called chymopapase.

Paresthesia. Peculiar symptoms termed tingling, burning, prickling, pulling, or tightness. Usually indicates pressure on a nerve.

Peripheral nerve. A nerve outside the spinal column descending the arm or leg. These nerves carry sensation, transmit pain, and initiate muscle function.

Posterior. Behind; to the rear.

Posture. The appearance of a person standing erect with good balance and minimal effort.

Prolapsed disk. Herniated, bulging, or ruptured disk.

Prone position. A person lying face down on stomach.

Psychosomatic pain. A pain perceived by the patient that has no apparent discernible organic cause.

Radicle. Nerve root.

Radiculitis. Inflammation of a radicle, causing pain or paresthesia in the distribution of a dermatome or myotome.

Ruptured disk. Herniated, bulging, or protruding disk. Implies protrusion of tissue through an abnormal opening.

Sacrum. The small bone within the pelvis at the base of the spinal column upon which is balanced the entire spinal column. At its tip is located the coccyx.

Sacroiliac joints. The two joints on each side of the sacrum that connect to the ilia of the pelvis.

Sciatic nerve. A large nerve formed by numerous nerves of the cord (L_4, L_5, S_1, S_2) that becomes united into one major nerve within the pelvis, then goes down the posterior portion of the thigh to the knee.

Slipped disk. A lay term similar to ruptured, bulging, or herniated disk.

Spinal canal. The opening in the center of the spine through which course the spinal cord and cauda equina.

Spinal cord. The major portion of the central nervous system going down from the brain to the thoracolumbar spine, where it divides to form the cauda equina.

Spinal column. Vertebral column. This is the spine, made up of seven (7) cervical vertebrae, twelve (12) thoracic vertebrae, five (5) lumbar vertebrae, and the sacrum-coccyx and their disks.

Straight leg raising test. This test, abbreviated S.L.R., indicates the presence of pressure on, or irritation of, the sciatic nerve roots when the leg is raised (flexed) with the knee straight. The test can be done by straightening the knee *after* the hip has been flexed to 90 degrees. A positive test indicates that there is pain doing this test, which means there is a nerve pressure or irritation.

Stenosis. Narrowing. Spinal stenosis means a narrowing of the spinal canal.

Supine position. The position of a person lying on his or her back, face up.

Syndrome. A group of symptoms or signs that are all related to one cause or one disease.

Thoracic spine. The twelve (12) vertebrae above the lumbar spine and below the cervical spine. The thoracic spine humps, or forms a kyphosis.

Trauma. An injury, usually physical but may be psychological.

Tumor. Any growth or enlargement, not necessarily cancer but larger than normal.

Vertebra; Vertebrae (plural). The individual bones that make up the spine.

Vertebral column. The spinal column. This is the spine, made up of seven (7) cervical vertebrae, twelve (12) thoracic vertebrae, five (5) lumbar vertebrae, and the sacrum-coccyx and their disks.

Vertebral disk. One of the disks between each pair of vertebrae throughout the spinal column.

Index

An italic number following an entry indicates an illustration.

pain in
    improper bending and, 62–71
    improper lifting and, 62–71
  relaxation of
    exercise for, *128*
  rotary stretch of, 115–117, *116, 117*
muscles of, 9, *32*, 51
  bending and, *34*
  function of, 51
  mental control of, *38*
  pain and, 51
proper use of, 142
re-extension of, proper, 143–144, *143*
stretching of, by traction, 131–133
support of, with corset, 134–135
sway
  as cause of pain, reason for, *95*
  back pain and, 52
Back injury
  distractions causing, 147
  from unexpected step, *74*
  low
    improper lifting and, 145–146, *146*
    most common cause of, 145
Back muscles(s), elongation of, 174–175
  relaxation of, 174–175
Back pain
  cancer as cause of, 156
  functional unit and, arching of, 56
  in deconditioned individual, 62–63
  in tense person, 72–73
  low
    arthritis as cause of, 157
    causes of, summary of, 173
    chronic, 168–172
      acupuncture in, 171, *172*
      biofeedback in, 170
      drugs for, 171
      imagery therapy in, 170
      progressive relaxation and, 170–171
      psychotherapy for, 172
      secondary gains from, 169
      TENS in, 169–170
      treatment of, 169
    degenerative arthritis as cause of, 161
    excessive lordosis and, 54–55
    fiber shortening and, 63
    from poor posture, 52–61
    high heels and, 56–57
    leg pain with, ruptured disk and, 76–89
    lordotic posture and, 63
    manipulation and, 136–140

  mechanical, 3–4
  nerve compression and, 56
  postural, observation of, 56
  psychological aspects of, 162–167
    secondary gains and, 163
    tertiary gains and, 164
  recurrent, 106
  sciatic nerve roots and, 45–46
  sites of, 43
  special causes of, 154–161
  treatment of, 106–147
    essentials for, *108*
  types of, 52
  unusual activities and, 72–75
  muscle spasm as cause of, 58–59
  sneezing and, 72, *73*
  while returning to erect posture, 64–67
  with leg pain, 57–58
  without leg pain, 57–58
Back school, 142
Back spasm, with sciatica, 86–87
Back surgery, failure of, 153
Backache
  avoidance of, proper sitting positions and, 54
  effect of gravity on, 107
  from excessive arching, 52
  from faulty sitting positions, 54
  from faulty sleeping habits, 53–54
  low
    acute, 106
      bed rest for, 107
      treatment for, 107
    chronic, 106, 147
    faulty sitting positions and, *58*
    predominant factors in, summary of, 174
    recurrent, 140
    relief of, time for, 109
    sagging mattress and, 57
   prolonged standing and, *56*
Backbone. *See* Spine.
Balance, spinal, *27*, 29
Bamboo spine, 157
Beach ball action, of disk nucleus, 16, *16*
Bed rest
  for acute low backache, 107
  positioning for, 107
Bending, 41
  acceptable twisting during, 41–42
  improper, *66*, 141
    distractions causing, *67*
    low back pain from, 62–71

188

MALIGNANCY(IES), low back pain and, 3
Malingering, 169
Manipulation
    contraindications to, 137
    for low back pain, 136–140
    functional unit and, 137–138
    pain relief and, 138–139
    repeated, other forms of treatment and,
        139
    return of spasm after, 139
    rotatory, *138*
    spinal flexibility and, 139–140
    techniques of, 136–137
    unlocking joints with, 139
Marie-Strumpell rheumatoid spondylitis,
        157
Marrow, contents of, 7–8
Massage, for low back pain, 112–113
Mechanical stress, vs. tearing of annulus,
        58
Mental control
    of back muscles, *38*
    of bending, 35–40
Mental status, low back pain and, 63
Metrizamide, 179
    for myelogram, 101–102
Military posture, back pain from, 52, 55
Minnesota Multiphasic Personality Inven-
        tory (M.M.P.I.), 165–167, *166*
    validity scales in, 167
Modality
    definition of, 169
    treatment, 169
Mopping, proper, diagonal principle of,
        145
Movement(s)
    limitation of, pain and, location of, 175
    proper, as habit, 146–147
Mucopolysaccharide, 179
Muscle(s)
    abdominal
        gravity and, 120–121
        oblique, exercises for, 122, *124*
        strong, need for, in exercises, 118–121
    back, 9, 51
        bending and, *34*
        elongation of, 174–175
        function of, 51
        mental control of, *38*
        pain and, 51
        relaxation of, 174–175
        sensor tissues of, 30, *31*

contraction, recording of, 103
erector, 9
erector spinae, *32*, 51
    pain and, 51
extensor, spinal movement and, 129, *130*
extensor hallucis longus, 81
gluteus maximus, *32*
hamstring, flexibility of 63
lazy, use of corset and, 135
oblique abdominalis, *32*
quadratus lumborum, *32*
spinal bending and, control of, 30–31,
        31, *32*
strengthened, making use of, 141–142
stretching of, manipulation and, 138
thigh, 81–82
Muscle spasm, as cause of back pain, 58–59
    mechanism of pain in, 69
    sprain and, 59
    strain and, 59
    with sprain, 68
Muscle tone, corset and, 134
Muscle-tendon unit, 83–84
Myelogram, 101–102, *102*, 179
    lumbar, *102*
Myotome, 179

NERVE(S)
    compression of, low back pain and, 56
    damage to, sensation with, 49
    femoral
        radiculitis in, 87–89
        stretch test of, 88–89, *89*
    fifth lumbar, 80, *81*, *82*, 98
    first sacral, 80, *81*, 98
    fourth lumbar, 98
    irritation of, sensation with, 49
    lubrication of, by dura, 48
    peripheral, 180
    protection of, by dura, 48
    sciatic, 47, *79*, 180
        pain in, 77, *78*, *79*, 80
        roots of, 80–83, *81*, *82*
        stretching of, 85
            pain and, 84
    skin map of, *78*, 80
    tendons and, 84
    third lumbar, 98
    Type I, 139
    Type II, 139
    Type III, 139
Nerve pressure, 83

189

Psychological aspects, of low back pain, 162–167
Psychopathology, presence of, determination of, 166
Psychosomatic pain, 180
Psychotherapy, for chronic low back pain, 172

QUADRATUS lumborum muscle(s), 32

RADICLE(S), 80, 180
Radiculitis, 80, 180
  femoral nerve, 87–89
Raking, proper, diagonal principle of, 145
Recurrent low backache, 140
Re-extension, of spine, twisting during, 144
  proper, of back, 143–144, 143
Reflex(es)
  ankle, 177
  ankle jerk, 84
  knee, 179
    diminished, 87
  knee jerk, 84
  muscle-tendon units and, 83–84
  tendon, 85
Reflex hammer, 85
Relaxation, progressive, in treatment of low back pain, 170–171
Reverse isometric abdominal exercises, 122
Rheumatoid arthritis, as cause of low back pain, 157
Rhythm, lumbar-pelvic, 33–34
Root(s), nerve. See Nerve root(s).
Rotary stretch exercise(s), 115–117, 116, 117
Rotatory manipulation, 138
Running, vs. jogging, 140, 141
Ruptured disk, 75–89, 77, 180
  limited flexibility with, 88
  pain and, 175
  surgery on, 149, 150

SACROILIAC joint, 5, 180
Sacrum, 5, 180
  angle of, lumbar spine and, curvature of, 53
  rotation of, 34
  spinal balance and, 27
Salicylate(s), for arthritis, 161. See also Aspirin.
Sciatic nerve, 47, 180
  roots of, 80–83, 81, 82

Sciatic pain, sway back and, 95
Sciatic scoliosis, 87
Sciatica, 77, 78, 79, 80
  back spasm with, 86–87
  stretching of nerve and, 84
Scoliosis
  acute, 67, 69
    nerve root pressure and, 89
  functional, 26, 69
  sciatic, 87
  structural, 29
Secondary gain(s), from low back pain, 163, 169
Self-hypnosis, in treatment of low back pain, 170
Sensitive tissue. See Tissue(s), sensitive.
Sensory map, for localization of pain, 165
Sensory skin map, 78
Set(s), of exercises, 121
Sheath(s)
  back movement and, 35
  of muscles, 31
  of nerve roots, 48. See also Dura.
Shortening
  of back muscles, bending and, 34
  of fibers, back pain and, 63
Sitting position(s)
  faulty
    backache from, 54
    low backache and, 58
  from lying position, 111–112
  proper, to avoid backache, 54
Situp(s), with legs straight, reasons for not doing, 124–125, 125, 126
Sleeping habits, faulty, low back pain and, 53–54, 57
Slipped disk, 180
Sneezing, back stress and, 72, 73
Spasm
  as cause of pain, 75
  back, with sciatica, 86–87
  manipulation and, 139
  muscle, as cause of back pain, 58–59
  protective, 74
    inflammation and, 75
Spinal canal, 180
  nerve roots and, 46
  width of, measurement of, 102
Spinal column, 181
Spinal column stress, low back pain and, 72
Spinal cord, 181